A SELF-INSTRUCTIONAL GUIDE TO
ORAL SURGERY IN GENERAL DENTISTRY

edited by

James R. Hooley, DDS
Robert J. Whitacre, MS, DDS

CHAPTER THREE

MEDICATIONS USED IN ORAL SURGERY

(ISBN #0-89939-030-7)

by

James R. Hooley, DDS
Robert J. Whitacre, MS, DDS

A SELF-INSTRUCTIONAL GUIDE TO ORAL SURGERY IN GENERAL DENTISTRY

(Complete Series ISBN #0-89939-000-5)

edited by

JAMES R. HOOLEY, DDS

Chairman
Dept. of Oral & Maxillofacial Surgery
School of Dentistry
University of Washington
Seattle, Washington

ROBERT J. WHITACRE, MS, DDS

Assistant Director
Office of Instructional Development
School of Dentistry
University of Washington
Seattle, Washington

Chapter One — **Instruments Used for Oral Surgery**
(ISBN #0-89939-010-2)

Two — **The Removal of Teeth**
(ISBN #0-89939-020-X)

Three — **Medications Used in Oral Surgery**
(ISBN #0-89939-030-7)

Four — **Surgical Complications**
(ISBN #0-89939-040-4)

Five — **Asepsis in Oral Surgery (Dental Asepsis)**
(ISBN #0-89939-050-1)

Six — **Assessment of and Surgery for Impacted Mandibular Third Molars**
(ISBN #0-89939-060-9)

Seven — **Pre-Prosthetic Surgery**
(ISBN #0-89939-070-6)

Eight — **Principles of Biopsy**
(ISBN #0-89939-080-3)

Nine — **Diagnosis and Treatment of Odontogenic Infections**
(ISBN #0-89939-090-0)

published by

Stoma Press, Inc.

13231 42nd Avenue NE
Seattle, WA 98125
(206) 365-2665

Printed By

ATOMIC PRESS
1421 N 34th
Seattle, WA
(206) 632-0550

Typeset By

CASTEEL TYPESETTING
18316 1st NE
Seattle, WA 98155
(206) 363-9054

MEDICATIONS USED IN ORAL SURGERY

by

JAMES R. HOOLEY, DDS
Chairman
Dept. of Oral & Maxillofacial Surgery
School of Dentistry
University of Washington
Seattle, Washington

ROBERT J. WHITACRE, MS, DDS
Assistant Director
Office of Instructional Development
School of Dentistry
University of Washington
Seattle, Washington

CONSULTANTS

ERNEST W. SMALL, DDS, MS
Department of Oral and Maxillofacial Surgery
School of Dentistry
University of North Carolina
Chapel Hill, North Carolina

JAMES H. QUINN, DDS
Department of Oral and Maxillofacial Surgery
School of Dentistry
Louisiana State University
New Orleans, Louisiana

RALPH G. MERRILL, DDS, MScD
Chairman
THOMAS W. ALBERT, DMD, MD
J. THEODORE JASTAK, DDS, PhD
OSCAR N. LUCAS, DDS, PhD
Department of Oral and Maxillofacial Surgery
School of Dentistry
University of Oregon
Portland, Oregon

ROBERT A. MIDDLETON, DDS
Chairman
LUCIAN SZMYD, DMD, MS
Department of Oral Surgery
School of Dentistry
University of the Pacific
San Francisco, California

GORDON W. PEDERSEN, DDS, MSD
Department of Oral Surgery
School of Dentistry
Case-Western Reserve University
Cleveland, Ohio

RICHARD A. SMITH, DDS
Division of Oral Surgery
School of Dentistry
University of California
San Francisco, California

MARTIN S. LEBOWITZ, DDS, MS
Chairman
JEFFREY L. LASKIN, DDS, MS
Department of Oral Surgery
College of Dentistry
University of Florida
Gainsville, Florida

MONTY REITZIK, BDS, FDSRCS, MB, ChB
Department of Oral Surgery
Faculty of Dentistry
The University of British Columbia
Vancouver, Canada

B. K. ARORA, BDS, DMD, MS (Oral Surgery), **FRCD, FICD**
Chairman
Department of Oral Surgery and Anesthesia
College of Dentistry
University of Saskatchewan
Saskatoon, Canada

M. K. HAMILTON, DDS
Chairman
Department of Oral Surgery
School of Dentistry
University of Maryland
Baltimore, Maryland

GERALD R. OTT, DDS
Chairman
Department of Oral Surgery
College of Dentistry
University of Nebraska
Lincoln, Nebraska

DORAN E. RYAN, DDS, MS
Chairman
SIDNEY L. BRONSTEIN, DDS, MScD
Division of Oral Surgery
School of Dentistry
University of Colorado
Denver, Colorado

BERNARD C. BYRD, DDS, MS
Chairman
Department of Oral Surgery
School of Dentistry
Loma Linda University
Loma Linda, California

KIMBLE A. TRAEGER, DMD
RICHARD S. ALLEY, DDS, MSD
Department of Oral and Maxillofacial Surgery
The University of Texas Health Science Center at San Antonio
San Antonio, Texas

LAWRENCE SALMAN, DDS, MPA
Chairman
Department of Oral and Maxillofacial Surgery
College of Dentistry
New York University
New York, New York

RICHARD D. MALLOW, DDS, MS
RICHARD G. STAPLEFORD, DDS
Department of Oral Surgery
School of Dentistry
University of Detroit
Detroit, Michigan

PHILIP D. MARANO, DDS
Director
Department of Oral and Maxillofacial Surgery
School of Dentistry
Oral Roberts University
Tulsa, Oklahoma

ERIC P. MILLAR, DDS, FRCD, FICD
Associate Director
Division of Oral Surgery
Faculty of Dentistry
McGill University
Montreal, Quebec

LEON D. FIELDER, DDS
Chairman
MARTIN STEINER, DDS
Department of Oral and Maxillofacial Surgery
School of Dentistry
University of Louisville
Louisville, Kentucky

JOE HALL MORRIS, DDS
Chairman
HOWARD S. MISNER, DDS
Department of Oral and Maxillofacial Surgery
College of Dentistry
University of Tennessee
Memphis, Tennessee

KENNETH W. HUGHES, DDS
Department of Oral and Maxillofacial Surgery
College of Dentistry
University of Illinois
Chicago, Illinois

ALBERT F. STAPLES, DMD, PhD
Chairman
Department of Oral Surgery
College of Dentistry
University of Oklahoma
Oklahoma City, Oklahoma

LOUIS G. MERCURI, DDS, MS
Department of Oral and Maxillofacial Surgery
School of Dentistry
Medical College of Virginia / Virginia Commonwealth University
Richmond, Virginia

TABLE OF CONTENTS

Page

MESSAGE TO LEARNER 6
OVERVIEW AND OBJECTIVES 7
INTRODUCTION TO CHAPTER 9

UNIT I — FUNDAMENTALS OF PRESCRIBING MEDICATIONS 10
- Pre-Test—Unit I 10
- Introduction 12
- Parts of a prescription 12
- Posology (Drug Dosage) 17
- Latin Abbreviations 18

UNIT II — USE OF REFERENCES 19
- Pre-Test—Unit II 19
- Introduction 21
- Accepted Dental Therapeutics 21
- AMA Drug Evaluations 21
- U. S. Pharmacopeia Dispensing Information 22
- Physician's Desk Reference and Compendium of Pharmaceuticals and Specialties 23
- Dictionary of Drug Names 24

UNIT III — ANTIBIOTICS 26
- Pre-Test — Unit III 26
- Introduction 28
- Summary of Antibiotics Commonly Used in Dentistry 28
- Description of Antibiotics Commonly Used in Dentistry 28
  - PENICILLINS 28
    - Penicillin-G 29
    - Procaine Penicillin-G 29
    - Penicillin-V 30
    - Sodium Dicloxacillin 30
    - Ampicillin 30
  - ERYTHROMYCIN 32
  - TETRACYCLINES 33
  - CLINDAMYCIN AND LINCOMYCIN 34
  - CEPHALOSPORINS 35
  - AMINOGLYCOSIDES 36
- Prophylactic Use of Antibiotics 38
- Antibiotics and Their Usual Adult Dosages 40

12—

UNIT IV — ANALGESICS 41
Pre-Test—Unit IV 41
Introduction 44
Strategy for Post-Operative Analgesia 45
Mild Analgesics 46
ASPIRIN 46
IBUPROFEN 47
ACETAMINOPHEN 48
CODEINE 49
PROPOXYPHENE 50
Moderate Analgesics 51
CODEINE PLUS ASPIRIN 52
CODEINE PLUS ACETAMINOPHEN 52
Strong Analgesics 53
MEPERIDINE 53
PENTAZOCINE 54
OXYCODONE 55
Guidelines for Analgesic Use in Oral Surgery 56
Grouping of Analgesics by Relative Analgesic Effectiveness 56

SUMMARY OF REFERENCES AND LITERATURE CITED 59
USEFUL ADDITIONAL SOURCES OF INFORMATION 59
REVIEW OF LITERATURE PERTAINING TO PHENYLALKANOIC ACID DERIVATIVES (IBUPROFEN AND FENBUFEN) 60
SUMMARY OF ANTIBIOTIC PRESCRIPTIONS AND NOTES 61
SUMMARY OF ANALGESIC PRESCRIPTIONS AND NOTES 62
SUMMARY OF OTHER PRESCRIPTIONS AND NOTES 63

MESSAGE TO LEARNER

When reading a standard textbook, it is often difficult for you to know exactly what the important content is. It is difficult to separate areas that are essential for you to understand from those that are nice to know. You may often have thought you knew the material but could not apply it when presented with the clinical situation. You may also have had a problem during examinations when instructors asked you questions that were **not** covered in your reading.

In writing this chapter, considerable time and effort have been invested in creating a feedback system for you to monitor your learning progress. We have included a section termed "overview and objectives" which states the essential kinds of performances or knowledge you can expect to gain from reading the contents and completing the study exercises. Generally, we have included a **"Pre-Test"** for each unit. The "Pre-Test" is intended to show you what you don't know about the content of the unit. It is difficult for you to see learning take place unless you have both a "before" and "after" demonstration. You should retake the pre-tests following completion of each unit.

The **study exercises** are designed for different levels of learning. The **first level** of study exercises are of the "fill in the blank" type. The blanks usually include "key" words or phrases taken from the content preceding the study exercise.

The **second level** of study exercises is designed as problem-solving tasks. Generally these take a small piece of a larger concept and allow you to focus your attention on mastery of the piece. Learning one piece at a time is similar to learning your multiplication tables. The small pieces are then assimilated into larger concepts which you can learn with ease.

The **third level** of questions are simulations of clinical problems that you will be faced with in treating patients. Having completed the previous study exercises, you should be able to adequately cope with these. These are the most important study exercises because they resemble the real world of dentistry. Through adequate analysis and planning, complications or surprises during surgery can be greatly reduced. These are similar to "story problems" in mathematics.

The study exercises are **extremely important** and you should take the time to **write the answers** in the blanks or spaces provided. You may be tempted to mentally answer the questions or skip them entirely to save time. You will **retain more of the information** you have read with much **less effort** if you take the time to write out the answers as you proceed. Considerable research in self-instructional design and learning has shown the importance of answering such study questions.

Even though the content in these chapters appears large, by no means did we intend to present the entire field of oral surgery. We intend these chapters to be your "starter kit," and strongly encourage you to obtain other reference books, journals, and materials to cover topics not discussed.

Although we have had considerable input from many people in writing these chapters, we by no means imply that these techniques, instruments or concepts are the "only way." Your oral surgeon or instructors may wish to deviate from the methods described in these chapters — especially with regards to specific clinical situations.

OVERVIEW AND OBJECTIVES

This chapter presents a review of drugs most commonly used in dentistry for the treatment of infections and pain. It also reviews the fundamentals of prescribing medications and describes the use of accepted drug references. Potential drug interaction problems are also stressed.

WARNING: DO NOT USE ANY DRUGS WITHOUT FIRST CONSULTING ACCEPTED REFERENCE SOURCES.

UNIT I — FUNDAMENTALS OF PRESCRIBING MEDICATIONS

The purpose of Unit I, Fundamentals of Prescribing Medications, is for you to learn (or review) the components of a prescription and the format in which these components should be arranged.

Following completion of this unit, you will be able to:

1. Describe the function or purpose for the basic ten (10) components that should be included in any properly written prescription.
2. State the additional component required if you are prescribing narcotics.
3. Given the recommended adult drug dosage and the weight of a child, calculate by **Clark's Rule** the dosage that would be prescribed for the child. State a method to verify this dosage.
4. State **Young's Rule** and why it is not a good rule to follow when determining dosages for children.
5. Given the data for all necessary components of a prescription, correctly write the prescription.
6. Given an incorrectly prepared prescription, identify the deficiencies and state the consequences of the deficiencies.

UNIT II — USE OF REFERENCES

The purpose of this unit is for you to learn (or review) how to use standard pharmacological references as a basis for:

- Analyzing drugs your patient may be taking.
- Identifying potential drug interaction problems associated with your prescriptions.
- Verifying drug dosages and commercially available formulations.
- Reviewing instructions to give your patients.
- Verifying indications and contraindications for drugs you may prescribe.

Following completion of this unit you will:

1. State advantages and disadvantages for each of the six references listed below.
   a. ADT
   b. AMA Drug Evaluations
   c. USPDI
   d. PDR
   e. CPS
   f. Dictionary of Drug Names
2. Select the best reference for instructions for your patients.
3. Given a clinical situation requiring use of a drug reference, select the best reference from the six discussed in this unit.
4. State which two references have a section illustrating various drugs in color.
5. From the six references listed in this unit, select the one most useful for information on drug interactions.

UNIT III — ANTIBIOTICS

The purpose of this unit is for you to learn the indications and contraindications for prescribing the antibiotics presented in the unit. At the completion of this unit, you will:

1. State seven (7) indications for prophylactic use of antibiotics prior to dental treatment.
2. State the "first-line" drug of choice when treating a dental infection if you have no laboratory data (e.g., culture results and susceptibility tests).
3. State the drug of choice as an alternative to penicillin when your patient is allergic to penicillin.
4. State the general indications for use of the following drugs:
   a. Cephalosporins
   b. Aminoglycosides
   c. Tetracyclines
   d. Penicillins
   e. Erythromycin
   f. Clindamycin & Lincomycin
5. For each of the drugs listed in the previous objective, list the common adverse reaction(s).
6. For the penicillins below, state whether it is best used orally or IV:
   a. Penicillin G
   b. Penicillin V
7. State the penicillin(s) to prescribe if the infective organisms produce penicillinase.
8. Choose the appropriate regimen(s) for prophylactic antibiotics for each of the seven indications listed in objective 1 above.

UNIT IV — ANALGESICS

The purpose of this unit is for you to learn (or review) the important factors to consider when you use analgesics. Major guidelines, specific information concerning various anticipated pain levels and specific information concerning the different drugs commonly available are presented so that you may become more proficient in managing the problems of pain control. Following completion of this unit, you will:

1. State three (3) general guidelines for the use of analgesics.

2. Given this chapter as a reference source, write a prescription for each of the following nine (9) analgesics.

   a. Aspirin
   b. Ibuprofen
   c. Acetaminophen
   d. Codeine
   e. Propoxyphene
   f. Meperidine
   g. Pentazocine
   h. Oxycodone
   i. Combinations of codeine and other analgesics

3. State the advantages and disadvantages for the following nine (9) analgesics.

   a. Aspirin
   b. Ibuprofen
   c. Acetaminophen
   d. Codeine
   e. Propoxyphene
   f. Meperidine
   g. Pentazocine
   h. Oxycodone
   i. Combinations of codeine and other analgesics

4. Prescribe an appropriate analgesic from pain Groups I-III for a given clinical procedure.

5. Given a clinical situation in which you prescribed what you thought to be an adequate analgesic without success, describe your course of action.

INTRODUCTION TO MEDICATIONS USED IN ORAL SURGERY

Dentists are writing more prescriptions for drugs and medications now than in the past. Antibiotics and analgesics are by far the most frequently prescribed medications by dentists. Dentists in practice less than 5 years write more prescriptions than those having practiced more than 10 years. While physicians confer regularly with a pharmacist, dentists confer less often.[1]

With the increased use of drugs in society today, it becomes most important for dentists to have the background knowledge enabling them to:

1. Write a correct prescription.

2. Use the most up-to-date references for evaluation of the interaction between a patient's medications and planned dental therapy.

3. Select appropriate antibiotics for treatment of dental infections.

4. Select appropriate analgesics for the control of dental pain.

We have limited this chapter to the above topics. We have avoided trying to include descriptions of the wide variety of drug trade names, and instead stress the use of a relatively small group of generic drugs.

---

[1] ____________________ A Look at Prescriptions Dentists Write, Dental Economics, Oct. 1979, pp. 69-72.

Unit I

FUNDAMENTALS OF PRESCRIBING MEDICATIONS

Introduction
Parts of Prescription
Posology (Drug dosage)
Latin Abbreviations

PRETEST

- Answer the following questions.
- Compare your responses with the correct responses given on page 11.
- If all responses were correct, proceed to Unit II.
- If only some responses were correct, proceed to Unit I, page 12.
- The numbers in parentheses refer to the specific objective number from which the question was derived.

QUESTIONS

1. *Which of the items listed in question 2 are **required by law** to be on your prescription when you prescribe a Schedule II drug (03-01-01)?*

2. *Which of the items listed below are **commonly included** when writing any prescription (03-01-02)?*

   a. Date
   b. Patient's name
   c. Patient's address
   d. Doctor's name
   e. Doctor's address
   f. Patient's age
   g. Patient's weight
   h. Inscription
   i. Subscription
   j. Superscription
   k. ℞
   l. Signatura
   m. Signature
   n. DEA number
   o. BNDD number
   p. Dental license number
   q. Refill information
   r. Generic substitution information

3. *Clark's Rule is used to ____________________ (03-01-03).*

4. *Complete the following using Clark's rule (03-01-03):*

Drug	Adult Dose	Child Weight	Child Dose
a. Diazepam	15 mg	100 lbs	________
b. Pentobarbital	100 mg	20 lbs	________
c. Codeine	30 mg	50 lbs	________

5. *Young's rule calculates children's drug dosage on the basis of ____________. The formula is: Child dose = adult dose x ____________ (03-01-04)*

6. When calculating drug dosage for children, Clark's Rule is preferred over Young's Rule (03-01-04).

7. If you are prescribing a drug for a child (or a small adult) and you are unsure of the proper dosage, what should you do (03-01-03)? consult pharmacist

Critique the prescriptions below. Give the letter code from question #2 for any items not present or incorrectly filled out and state the consequences of this error (03-01-06).

8.

Barbara Evans, DDS

(No) Doctor's address

Name Mary Smith Date 7-26-82
Address 4386 122nd St. Age 23

℞ Meperidine (No) dosage
Dispense ten
Take one q 4-6 hr prn pain

No Refills
✓ Substitution permitted
___ Dispense as written

Barbara Evans D.D.S.

DEA # (No) DEA #

9.

Larry K. Morrison, DDS.
18316 - 1st N.E.
Missoula, Montana
556-1212

Date (not) complete

Name William Jones Date Aug. 16
Address 4830 Lincoln Ave. Age 24

℞ Percodan — better generically written
Dispense 8 — can be easily changed
Take 1 stat then 1 q 6 h prn pain

___ Refills — should be specified.
___ Substitution permitted — helps pharmacy if they don't have the same brand.
✓ Dispense as written

Larry K. Morrison D.D.S.

DEA # AM3762823

PRETEST ANSWERS

1. a, b, c, d, e, h, i, l, m, n
2. a, b, c, d, e, f, h, i, j, k, l, m, n, q, r
3. Calculate proper drug dosage for children based weight on weight.
4. a. 10 mg
   b. 20 mg
   c. 10 mg
5. Age, child's age ÷ (age + 12)
6. Clark's, Young's
7. Consult a pharmacist
8. e. Without a doctor's address, this cannot be filled.
   h. The dosage is not specified
   n. This prescription rquires a DEA number to be dispensed.
9. a. Without the date this cannot be filled.
   h. This would be better if written generically.
   i. Should be "eight." This could be changed to "18" or "80."
   q. It should specify whether or not refills are permitted.
   r. The pharmacy may not stock this brand and would not be able to substitute another.

Unit I

FUNDAMENTALS OF PRESCRIBING MEDICATIONS

INTRODUCTION

A prescription is an order to a pharmacist for dispensing a definite amount of a specific drug to a patient along with instructions on its use. Care should be taken in composing the prescription to minimize the possibilities of misinterpretation.

PARTS OF A PRESCRIPTION

A standard prescription format has been established which will assist you in providing the correct information to the pharmacist. This format is shown below and each item is discussed.

1. Dentist's name and office address
2. Date
3. Name and address of patient
4. Age
5. Superscription
6. Inscription
7. Subscription
8. Signatura
9. Refill information
10. Generic substitution
11. Dentist's signature
12. DEA #

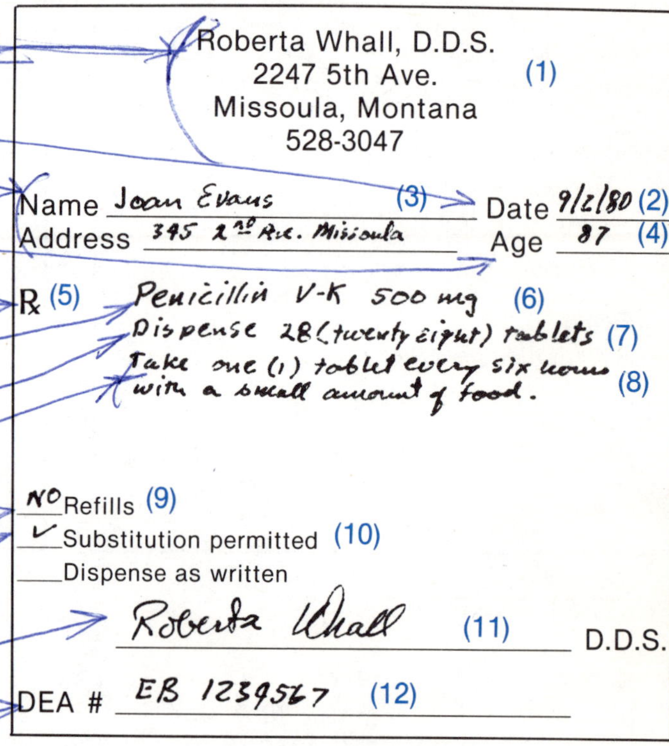

Roberta Whall, D.D.S.
2247 5th Ave. (1)
Missoula, Montana
528-3047

Name Joan Evans (3) Date 9/2/80 (2)
Address 345 2nd Ave. Missoula Age 87 (4)

℞ (5) Penicillin V-K 500 mg (6)
Dispense 28 (twenty eight) tablets (7)
Take one (1) tablet every six hours with a small amount of food. (8)

NO Refills (9)
✓ Substitution permitted (10)
___ Dispense as written

Roberta Whall (11) D.D.S.

DEA # EB 1239567 (12)

1. **Dentist's name and office address**

   Dentist's name and address is required by law. If it is not printed on your prescription blanks, you must write it in.

2. **Date**

   Since a prescription is a legal document, it must be dated. It is required by the Controlled Substances Act of 1970 that Schedule II drugs be dispensed by a pharmacist on the day the prescription is issued.

3. **Name and address of patient**

   As required by law, the address of the patient must be included in prescriptions for Schedule II drugs.

4. **Age** (Optional)

Stating your patient's age allows the pharmacist to detect errors in dosage, e.g., adult dose prescribed for a child.

5. **Superscription**

The sign ℞ preceding the prescription is termed the superscription. Some regard this sign as a sentimental gesture with no practical significance. The symbol "R" (without the x) represents the Latin word meaning "take thou." The small stroke placed across one leg of the R (as ℞) is of ancient derivation, a relic of the days when all prescriptions were prefaced by a prayer to the Roman god, Jupiter, invoking his blessing upon the efficacy of the medicine.

6. **Inscription**

The inscription is the place for the **name of the drug** and the **dosage form.** The **generic name** of a drug should be used, if possible, because:

- It is desirable to avoid using multiple names for the same drug to reduce the amount of memorization and possible confusion.
- By prescribing the generic form of drug, you give the pharmacist the option to dispense the least expensive brand.
- If you prescribe a drug by brand name and the pharmacy does not stock that particular brand, they will not be able to fill the prescription unless you specify that generic equivalent substitutions are acceptable. (Generic substitution may or may not be allowed in your state or province. You should review these regulations in your practice area.)

The **dosage form** for most tablets and capsules should be included since a drug may come in multiple dosage units, i.e., potassium penicillin-V is available in 500 mg, 250 mg, or 125 mg tablets. When prescribing a liquid, the dose of the drug per volume should be mentioned. However, there are exceptions to this rule. It is not necessary to write out the dosage of each of the component drugs in a proprietary such as Empirin Compound #3.

7. **Subscription**

The subscription is the quantity of medication to be dispensed. It is usually given as the total number of tablets or capsules or as the total volume to be dispensed. It is not the dosage for each administration. You should write the number of tablets in words as well as numerically to prevent anyone from altering the prescription. For example, if you write "10 tablets," it could be easily changed to "40 tablets." This could not be altered if written as "10 (ten) tablets."

8. **Signatura** (Instructions)

The signatura is the directions to the patient for how much to take at what time intervals. This information will be typed out by the pharmacist and usually included on the label of the prescription. It is wise to write this information out in cursive rather than using Latin abbreviations so there will be no misinterpretations. With experience, and especially if you find that you are writing a number of prescriptions, you may find it easier to use Latin abbreviations to shorten the procedure. These can be found in any reference book such as the American Dental Association's "Accepted Dental Therapeutics." The most common abbreviations are summarized on page 18 of this chapter.

9. **Refill information**

It is usually wise to place "no refill" on the prescription. This will force the patient to contact you if he or she feels a need for more of the drug than you prescribed.

10. **Generic substitution**

In many states, it is required by law that you specify whether generically-equivalent substitution is permitted. Unless you desire the placebo effect of a particular color or appearance of a drug, a generically-equivalent substitution will provide your patient with equal benefits and may enable the pharmacist to dispense a less expensive brand, or the brand they routinely stock.

11. **Dentist's signature**

The dentist's signature is required by law for Schedule II drugs. DO NOT have your signature printed on your prescription pads.

12. **Drug Enforcement Administration Registration Number** (DEA #)

This number is required only when prescribing Schedules II and III drugs as specified by the United States Controlled Substances Act of 1970. A similar number is required in most other countries. **This number should not be printed on your prescription pad.**

STUDY EXERCISE

Examine the following prescription. For each of the numbers in parentheses:

a. Give the name of this part of the prescription.
b. State the reason or purpose for this information.
c. State whether this part of the prescription is written correctly.
d. State the consequence if not correctly filled out.

Larry K. Morrison, D.D.S.
(1) 18316 - 1st N.E.
Missoula, Montana
556-1212

Name William Jones — Date Aug. 16 (2)
Address 4830 Lincoln Ave. — Age 24

(3) ℞ (4) Oxycodone HCl 5 mg plus Acetaminophen 325 mg
(5) Dispense 5
(6) Take 1 stat then 1 q 6 h prn pain

No Refills
✓ Substitution permitted
___ Dispense as written

(7) Larry K Morrison, D.D.S.
(8) D.E.A. # ________

ANSWERS

1. a. Prescriber's name and address
   b. Required by law
   c. Correct
   d. Prescription is unfillable if this portion is not completed

2. a. Date
   b. Required by law if prescribing Schedule II drug
   c. Incorrect. Year is missing
   d. Prescription cannot be filled

3. a. Superscription
   b. Customary symbol
   c. Correct

4. a. Inscription
   b. Drug name and dose
   c. Correct brand name

5. a. Subscription
   b. Designates how much medication is to be dispensed
   c. Incorrect. The number should be written in words.
   d. As written, this prescription could be altered to "dispense 50." This error is especially dangerous when prescribing narcotics.

6. a. Signatura
   b. Directions to be typed on label
   c. Correct. This illustrates the use of Latin abbreviations.

7. a. Signature
   b. Required by law
   c. Correct. Signature should not be printed on blank prescription pads

8. a. DEA #
   b. Required by law when prescribing Schedule II drugs
   c. Incorrect
   d. Without a DEA # this narcotic prescription cannot legally be filled

For the following situations, select the pertinent data and complete a blank prescription below. Your DEA number is EB-8782431. For each, substitutions permitted, no refills.

9. Sally Doe, 2239 N. Seneca St., 42 year-old female, 130 lbs., Codeine Sulfate, 30 mg tablets, 10 tablets. Take one tablet q 3 h prn pain.

10. Jim Shue, 506 Stewart, Apt. B, 23-year-old male, 150 lbs., Erythomycin Stearate, 250 mg tablets, 28 tablets. Take one tablet every 6 hours for seven days.

Barbara Evans, D.D.S.
18316 1st Ave. E.
San Francisco, California
228-4242

Name SALLY DOE Date 10-10-82
Address 2239 N, SENECA ST. Age 42

℞ CODEINE SULFATE, 30 mg.
DISP. 10 TABS (TEN)
1 TAB q 3 h PRN PAIN

NO Refills
✓ Substitution permitted
____ Dispense as written

____________ D.D.S.

DEA # EB 8782431

Barbara Evans, DDS
18316 1st Ave. E.
San Francisco, California
228-4242

Name JIM SHUE Date 10-10-82
Address 506 STEWART, APT. B Age 23

℞ ERYTHROMYCIN STEARATE, 250 mg
DISP. 28 TABS. (TWENTY-EIGHT)
1 TAB q 6 h FOR 7 DAYS.

NO Refills
✓ Substitution permitted
____ Dispense as written

____________ D.D.S.

DEA # EB-8782431

9.

Barbara Evans, D.D.S.
18316 - 1st Ave. E.
San Francisco, California
228-4242

Name Sally Doe Date Today's Date
Address 2239 N. Seneca St. Age 42

℞ Codeine Sulfate 30 mg
Dispense 10 (ten) tablets
Take one tablet q 3 h prn pain

No Refills
✓ Substitution permitted
___ Dispense as written

Barbara Evans, D.D.S.
D.E.A. # #EB 8782431

10.

Barbara Evans, D.D.S.
18316 - 1st Ave. E.
San Francisco, California
228-4242

Name Jim Shue Date Today's Date
Address 506 Stewart Apt. B Age 23

℞ Erythromycin Stearate 250 mg
Dispense 28 (twenty-eight) tablets
Take one tablet every six hours for seven days

No Refills
✓ Substitution permitted
___ Dispense as written

Barbara Evans, D.D.S.
D.E.A. # ___

POSOLOGY (Drug dosage)

The dosage for most drugs used in dentistry can be found by consulting "Accepted Dental Therapeutics" (ADT) and, less often, the Physician's Desk Reference (PDR) and United States Pharmacopeia Dispensing Information (USPDI).

Determining dosages for children can be a problem, especially when the medication comes in liquid form. ONE ACCEPTED METHOD IS THE USE OF A DOSE PER WEIGHT WHICH CAN SOMETIMES BE FOUND IN THE REFERENCE SOURCES. Unfortunately, there are still drugs for which this information is not available. A practical method to determine children's dosage (up to 16 years old) is **Clark's Rule,** which is:

$$\textbf{Clark's Rule: Child's dose} = \textbf{Adult dose} \times \frac{\textbf{Weight of child in pounds}}{\textbf{150 lbs.}}$$

Another historical method for determining child's dosage is **Young's Rule** which is:

$$\textbf{Young's Rule: Child dose} = \textbf{Adult dose} \times \frac{\textbf{Child's age}}{\textbf{Child's age + 12}}$$

This is not as good as Clark's Rule because drug action is more closely related to size (weight, volume or surface area) than age.

Neither of these rules is ideal for all cases. For example, penicillin should be prescribed in adult doses whatever the age or weight of the child. A good drug reference will specify children's dosage (or a method for calculating them). **If you are unsure of the proper dosage for children, you should consult your pharmacist for assistance.**

STUDY EXERCISE

Clark's Rule is used to determine drug dosages for children. It states that:

Child's Dose = ADULT DOSE x $\frac{\text{CHILD'S WEIGHT (lb's)}}{\textit{150 lbs}}$

Young's Rule states that: Child's Dose = ADULT DOSE x $\frac{\text{CHILD'S AGE}}{\text{CHILD'S AGE +12}}$

Use Clark's Rule to complete the following:

	Adult Dose	*Child Weight*	*Child Dose*
a.	*600,000 units*	*50 lb.*	200000
b.	*250 mg*	*30 lb.*	50
c.	*325 mg*	*75 lb.*	163
d.	*300,000 units*	*50 lb.*	100000

When computing a child's dose for a drug, CLARK'S *Rule is better than* Young's *Rule. If you are unsure of the proper dose, you should* CONSULT PHARMACIST.

ANSWERS

$$\text{Clark's Rule : Child's Dose} = \text{Adult Dose} \times \frac{\text{Weight in pounds}}{\text{150 pounds}}$$

$$\text{Young's Rule : Child's Dose} = \text{Adult Dose} \; \frac{\text{Age}}{\text{Age} + 12}$$

a. 200,000 units *b. 50 mg.* *c. 163 mg.* *d. 100,000 units*

When computing a child's dose Clark's Rule is better than Young's Rule. If you are unsure of the proper dose you should consult a pharmacist.

LATIN ABBREVIATIONS

The following Latin abbreviations are for your use as reference. With use, you will remember many of them.

Word, Phrase and Contraction	**Meaning**
aa (ana)	of each
a.c. (ante cibum)	before meals
p.c. (post cibum)	after meals
ad	up to
aq. (aqua)	water
f. (fac)	make
ft. (fiat)	let be made
h.s. (hora somni)	at bedtime
m. (misce)	mix
p.r.n. (pro re nata)	when needed
q.h. (quaque hora)	every hour
q. 2 h. (quaque secunda hora)	every two hours
q. 3 h. (quaque tertia hora)	every three hours
q. 4 h. (quaque quarta hora)	every four hours
q.s. (quantum sufficit)	a sufficient quantity
t.i.d. (ter in die)	three times a day
b.i.d. (bis in die)	twice a day
q.i.d. (quater in die) = q6h	four times a day
sig. (signa)	label (you write)
non rep. (ne repetatur)	do not repeat
ss. (semis)	one half
stat. (statim)	immediately

ī .... ONE

īī .... TWO

Unit II

USE OF REFERENCES

Introduction
Accepted Dental Therapeutics (ADT)
AMA Drug Evaluations
United States Pharmacopeia Dispensing Information (USPDI)
Physicians Desk Reference (PDR)
Compendium of Pharmaceuticals and Specialties (CPS)
Dictionary of Drug Names

PRETEST

- Answer the following questions.
- Compare your responses with the correct responses given.
- If all responses were correct, proceed to Unit III.
- If only some responses were correct, proceed to Unit II, page 21.
- The numbers in parentheses refer to the specific objective number from which the question was derived.

QUESTIONS

1. *List three acceptable references for drugs used in dentistry (03-02-03).*
   a. PDR
   b. ADT
   c. USPDI

2. *What are two disadvantages of the ADT as a reference for prescribing dental medications (03-02-01)?*
   a. ONLY DENTAL DRUGS.
   b. DEPTH OF DISCUSSION MAY BE INADEQUATE

3. *What reference would be especially useful if you want to provide your patients with easily understood instructions and precautions concerning a particular drug (03-02-02)?* USPDI — DISCUSSES IN LAY LANGUAGE

4. *The information in the* PDR or CPS *is provided by drug manufacturers while the information in the* ________ AMA Drug EVALUATIONS *is compiled by physicians and pharmacologists (03-02-01).*

5. Which of the following references would be the best source for dosage and drug interaction information (03-02-05; 03-02-03)?
   a. Physicians Desk Reference
   b. AMA Drug Evaluations
   c. Compendium of Pharmaceuticals and Specialties

6. While evaluating the health history of a new patient, you discover he is taking medication every 6 hours but does not know what the drug is or why it was prescribed. However, he does have 2 tablets with him. What reference might help you identify this drug (03-02-04; 03-02-03)? PDR or CPS — have color references

7. State the reference that would be the quickest source for a generic name if your patient only knows the trade name of her prescription (03-02-01). Dictionary of Drug Names.

ANSWERS

1. AMA Drug Evaluations
   Physicians Desk Reference
   U. S. Pharmacopeia Dispensing Information
   Accepted Dental Therapeutics
   Compendium of Pharmaceuticals and Specialties
   Dictionary of Drug Names

2. a. It includes only drugs used in dentistry.
   b. Depth of discussion may be inadequate.

3. USPDI — This reference includes discussions of medications in lay language.

4. PDR or CPS
   AMA Drug Evaluations

5. b

6. PDR or CPS — Both references include a section illustrating many tablets and capsules in color.

7. Dictionary of Drug Names

Unit II

USE OF REFERENCES

INTRODUCTION

With the hundreds of drugs in common usage, it will be impossible for you to memorize or remember all of the trade names, generic names, and specific dosages used in both medicine and dentistry. It will be necessary during your practicing career to have ready access to up-to-date reference materials. The five references chosen have different formats, advantages and disadvantages, thus some instruction is necessary to help you quickly obtain the information you need. The references below have been selected for specific content, depth, and applicability in dentistry.

- Accepted Dental Therapeutics (ADT)
- AMA Drug Evaluations
- United States Pharmacopeia Dispensing Information (USPDI)
- Physicians Desk Reference (PDR) (U.S.A.)
- Compendium of Pharmaceuticals and Specialties (CPS) (Canada)
- Dictionary of Drug Names

Each will be presented in terms of specific advantages. Understanding how and when to use each reference should save you valuable office time and reduce the possibilities for medical complications.

- **Accepted Dental Therapeutics**

This is the easiest to use of the reference sources for drugs common in dentistry. The ADT lists drugs by therapeutic use in the Table of Contents and by generic and trade names in two indexes. The actions, indications, contraindications, adverse reactions, precautions and dosage for each drug are listed.

Limitations of the ADT include:

- Its inclusion of only those drugs commonly used in dentistry.
- The depth of discussion may be inadequate for your needs.

The American Dental Association Council on Dental Therapeutics revises the ADT every two years. In view of rapid developments in this field, we recommend you purchase each edition as it becomes available.

- **AMA Drug Evaluations**

This reference source is revised periodically — usually every three years. It is a joint effort of the American Medical Association's Department of Drugs and the American Society for Clinical Pharmacology and Therapeutics.

It provides an excellent, easy-to-read, concise, and objective evaluation of drugs. It is much more comprehensive in scope than the ADT and more objective than the PDR or CPS. It also contains dispensing information and therefore might be a substitute for the PDR if you desire to purchase only one additional reference book (which we do not recommend).

- **United States Pharmacopeia Dispensing Information (USPDI)**

  This highly authoritative and inexpensive book is divided into two sections. The first contains dispensing information for almost every drug available, arranged alphabetically according to the generic name of the principal ingredient. The Advice to Patient section is the second section. It has information on each drug written in lay language. This information can easily be provided to your patients when it would be of benefit. Thus, the patient would have written instructions on the important precautions to follow, major drug interactions, and the precise method of taking the medication, e.g., one hour after meals, etc.

  The first section uses the following format:

  - Precautions to follow
  - Side effects
  - Patient consultation
  - General dosing information
  - Oral dosage forms

  This book does not contain information on the basic pharmacology of the drugs. It assumes the knowledge of basic pharmacology and therapeutics. Once the clinician knows what medication is indicated for the patient, there is no better reference for precautions, drug interactions and usual dosage forms. This book is updated every two months in the form of a newsletter.

  It is the easiest of all references to use since it uses only generic names. When using this reference, it becomes clear that one needn't get bogged down using trade names of drugs when it is so much easier to confine one's learning to generic names.

STUDY EXERCISES

1. The Accepted Dental Therapeutics is published by the American Dental Association and includes drugs commonly used in Dentistry.

2. List two disadvantages of the ADT.
   a. Easiest dental source to use.
   b. Lists drugs by therapeutic use

3. United States Pharmacopeia Dispensing Info. is a useful reference to use when providing your patients with instructions concerning a drug you have prescribed.

4. AMA Drug Evaluations provides a concise objective evaluation of drugs which is more comprehensive than the ADT.

- **Physicians Desk Reference (PDR) (USA)** or **Compendium of Pharmaceuticals and Specialties (CPS) (Used in Canada)**

The PDR (CPS) contains a description of about 2500 products. It is a confusing but useful book. It is provided free to physicians annually — but other health professionals must purchase it.

The PDR (CPS) is most useful when you must use trade names since all information is arranged alphabetically according to trade names. This is frequently necessary since most patients know only the trade name of the medications they are taking.

Perhaps the best use of this book is as an aid to history taking since the drugs can be identified and looked up in the PDR (CPS). However, for other information such as **dosage, drug interactions,** etc., the other books on the reference list are recommended over the PDR (CPS). All information in the PDR is provided by the drug manufacturers, not by physicians or pharmacologists.

The PDR is divided into seven sections. Listed in order of their appearance in the book, they are:

Section 1 (white) — Manufacturers' Index

Section 2 (pink) — Product Name Index
You will find a number following the product name. This number refers to the location in the white section, or Product Information Section, where you can find the description of the product.

Section 3 (blue) — Product Classification Index
This section lists products according to their general class of action (i.e., analgesics, anti-inflammatory agents, etc.). The classification is made by either the manufacturer or the publisher of the PDR.

Section 4 (yellow) — Generic and Chemical Name Index
In this section the products described in Product Information are listed under generic and chemical name headings according to the principle ingredients of the product.

Section 5 — Product Identification
This section presents actual-size color photographs of over 1,000 capsules and tablets. They are grouped by manufacturer. This section can be very helpful in identifying the "pills" your patient may bring to your office and in determining the medical problem associated with the patient's medication.

Section 6 (white) — Product Information
This is an alphabetical listing of products arranged by manufacturers in which the manufacturer describes the characteristics of the product.

Section 7 (green) — Diagnostic Products Information
This lists diagnostic products rather than pharmaceutical agents in alphabetical order by manufacturer. This section has limited use in dentistry at the present time.

The CPS is arranged in a similar fashion and contains similar information. The advantages and limitations of the CPS are similar to the PDR.

The **advantages** of the PDR and CPS include:

- The principal advantage of the PDR and CPS lies with their emphasis on the therapeutic use of drugs.
- An excellent cross-reference system. The drugs are most easily found when the trade name is known. The generic name can be found by first looking up the trade name. When only the generic name is known, the trade name can usually, but not always, be found.
- Very complete dosage information.
- Color illustrations of the most commonly prescribed drugs are provided and are frequently useful when health history information reveals your patient is taking "pills" for a medical problem and does not know the name of the drug, but has some capsules.

The **disadvantages** of the PDR and CPS include:

- The full disclosure of drug information (required by government agencies) frequently does not reflect the clinical use of the drugs.
- Descriptions of drugs are written by the manufacturer and are less objective than descriptions written by professional organizations such as the American Medical Association (AMA Drug Evaluations)
- The format is somewhat awkward to use in that it lists drugs by trade names from each manufacturer.

STUDY EXERCISES

1. The information in the PDR is provided by THE MANUFACTURER *and is, therefore, (more/less) ______ objective than information in the AMA Evaluations.*

2. Which of the following references might help you identify capsules your patient is taking? ______
a. PDR   b. ADT   c. AMA Drug Evaluations   d. CPS

3. ______ is most useful when the generic name of a drug is known.
a. USPDI   b. PDR   c. CPS

- **Dictionary of Drug Names**

The Dictionary of Drug Names is a listing of drugs by both trade names and generic names. This reference will enable you to look up the generic name from the trade names, therefore enabling you to look up the generic name in the USPDI. This book is published by The United States Pharmacopeial Convention with the first edition published in 1980. It is updated annually. You will find using the Dictionary of Drug Names in conjunction with the USPDI to be more convenient, more up to date and more clinically relevant than the PDR.

For each situation described below, state which of the references discussed in this chapter would be most useful.

4. *You have just prescribed a sedative for one of your pediatric patients. The patient's father wants you to explain the drug and any side effects or drug interactions which it might cause.* USPDI

5. *While taking a health history, you discover your patient is taking Robitet. She cannot tell you what the medication is or why she is taking it. You need to evaluate this drug.* PDR (CPS)

6. *You plan to write a prescription for fluoride supplements for a child who lives in a non-fluoridated area and you have forgotten the proper dosage for a 12-month-old child.* ADT

7. *An elderly patient cannot tell you what medications she is taking. However, she does keep several tablets in her purse. You need to identify these pink tablets.* PDR (CPS)

8. *You have just completed an extraction and plan to prescribe codeine for post-operative pain. You do not remember the proper dosage for adults.* ADT

9. *You want an unbiased evaluation of a new drug.* AMA Drug Evaluations

10. *You don't have a PDR and a patient tells you she is taking Motrin. You want to know the generic name so you can use the AMA evaluations to analyze it.* Dictionary of Drug Names.

ANSWERS

1. *Drug manufacturers, less*
2. *a, d*
3. *a*
4. *The USPDI would provide a description of the drug in lay language, which should answer the father's questions.*
5. *Both the PDR and the CPS list drugs by brand name. They would tell you what generic drug this is. Then, if you want detailed information about the drug action, you could consult the AMA Evaluations.*
6. *The ADT would be a quick, easy reference for this problem since fluoride supplements are drugs often used in dentistry.*
7. *The PDR and CPS have a section with colored illustrations of many drugs. You might be able to identify this drug by comparing it to these pictures.*
8. *Codeine is often used for dental pain and would be easily found in the ADT.*
9. *The AMA Drug Evaluations or USPDI would be the best sources. Both the PDR and CPS are published by drug manufacturers, while the AMA Drug Evaluations and USPDI are compiled by physicians and pharmacologists.*
10. *The Dictionary of Drug Names would be a quick, easy reference to find the generic name.*

Unit III

ANTIBIOTICS

Introduction
Prescribing Antibiotics
Antibiotics Commonly Used in Dentistry
Penicillins
Erythromycin
Tetracyclines
Clindamycin & Lincomycin
Cephalosporins
Aminoglycosides
Prophylactic Use of Antibiotics

PRETEST

- Answer the following questions.
- Compare your responses with the correct responses on page 27.
- If all responses are correct, proceed to Unit IV.
- If only some responses are correct, proceed to Unit III, page 28.
- The numbers in parentheses refer to the specific objective number from which the questions were derived.

QUESTIONS

1. *What is the antibiotic of choice for the treatment of nonspecific oral infections when a culture cannot be obtained (03-03-02)?* PENICILLIN - V

2. *What are the advantages and disadvantages of oral penicillin-G as opposed to penicillin-V (03-03-06)? Advantages:* BROADER RANGE OF EFFECT
Disadvantages: VARIABLY ABSORBED IN GI TRACT

3. *When is it appropriate to use sodium dicloxacillin (03-03-04)?*
VS. PENICILLINASE-PRODUCING STAPH.

4. *Why is tetracycline discouraged in the use for oral infections (03-03-05)?*
RESISTANCE OF STAPH. & STREP.

5. *When is clindamycin indicated in treating oral infections (03-03-04)?*
WHEN PENICILLINS CAN'T BE USED, & BACTERIA SENSITIVE TO CLINDAMYCIN

6. *When is erthromycin indicated in treating oral infections (03-03-03)?*
ALLERGIC TO PENICILLIN

7. *Since the cephalosporins are closely related to penicillins, should they be used when the patient has a history of penicillin allergy (03-03-05)?*
YES.

8. *When should an antibiotic be used prophylactically for any dental procedure (03-03-01)?*
   a. Rheumatic Fever
   b. Congenital Heart Valve Damage
   c. Valvular, Joint Prosthesis
   d. Steroid Therapy Recently
   e. Antineoplastic Therapy
   f. Disease which limits infection resistance

9. *If your patient comes to your office for treatment of an acute pulpitis but has a history of rheumatic fever, how would you manage the patient? (Include 3 alternative regimens.) (03-03-08)* Parenteral-Oral - Penicillin-G & Penicillin-V
   Oral - Penicillin-V
   Penicillin Allergy - Erythromycin

10. *Will you routinely prescribe Streptomycin, Gentamicin or Kenamycin in your office for treatment of oral infections in absence of gram strain or laboratory tests? Why or why not (03-03-05)?* No. — All are nephrotoxic & ototoxic

ANSWERS

1. Penicillin-V
2. Advantages: It has a broader effective range against bacteria.
   Disadvantages: It is variably absorbed in the G. I. tract.
3. When the bacteria have been shown to be penicillinase-producing staphylococci.
4. Because of the possible resistance of both streptococci and staphylococci to tetracycline.
5. Only when the bacteria involved have been shown to be sensitive to clindamycin and the penicillins cannot be used.
6. When penicillin is indicated and the patient is allergic to penicillin.
7. Yes, they can be used, but carefully.
8. Antibiotics should be used prophylactically only for patients with the following conditions:
   a. History of rheumatic fever or other diseases which predispose to valvular damage.
   b. Congenital valvular heart involvements.
   c. Valvular or other body prosthesis.
   d. Recent steroid therapy.
   e. Antineoplastic chemotherapy.
   f. History of a disease which limits the patient's ability to respond to infections (e.g., uncontrolled diabetes).
9. See page 38 of this chapter.
10. No. These drugs are nephrotoxic and ototoxic and should be used only when specifically indicated.

Unit III

ANTIBIOTICS

INTRODUCTION

The most commonly used antibiotics in dentistry will be presented along with short explanations of their use, dosages, and side effects. The use of antibiotics prophylactically will also be considered.

Prescribing Antibiotics

There is considerable debate about the proper use of antibiotics in dentistry. Many practitioners abuse these valuable medications through indiscriminate and unnecessary prescription writing. Because of the potential for selection of resistant organisms, antibiotics should only be prescribed when no other methods can be used to control infection. Whenever practical, culture and sensitivity testing should be performed to assure the use of the proper antimicrobial agent. You are referred to **Chapter 9, Diagnosis and Treatment of Odontogenic Infections** for more specific guidelines governing the use of antibiotics in clinical situations.

SUMMARY OF ANTIBIOTICS COMMONLY USED IN DENTISTRY

- Penicillins
  - ☐ Penicillin-G
  - ☐ Penicillin-V
  - ☐ Methicillin
  - ☐ Dicloxacillin
  - ☐ Ampicillin
- Erythromycin
- Tetracyclines
- Clindamycin & Lincomycin
- Cephalosporin
- Aminoglycosides

DESCRIPTION OF ANTIBIOTICS COMMONLY USED IN DENTISTRY

- **Penicillins**

The penicillins are the most useful and frequently prescribed antibiotics in dental use today. Though introduced for therapeutic use over thirty years ago, they have maintained their position as the primary antibiotic of choice for treatment of infections caused by oral flora (autogenous infections).

Penicillin is bacteriocidal against penicillin-sensitive microorganisms during the stage of active multiplication. It produces its effect by inhibiting biosynthesis of the cell wall. It is not active against bacteria producing penicillinase, which include many strains of staphylococci.

NOTE: Penicillin is still considered the "front line of treatment" for dental infections in the absence of culture and sensitivity data (see Chapter 9, Diagnosis and Treatment of Odontogenic Infections).

There are many different forms of penicillin available. These vary in their absorption, route of administration, and are effective against different bacterial species.

☐ Penicillin-G (Benzyl Penicillin)

There are many preparations of penicillin-G available. They differ only in their route of administration and duration of action.

Oral route — Oral penicillin-G is indicated in the treatment of mild to moderately severe infections caused by penicillin-G-sensitive microorganisms which are sensitive to the low serum levels common to this particular dosage form.

Since penicillin-G is destroyed by gastric acid, it should be administered one hour prior to meals or two hours after meals. Most clinicians find this to be a cumbersome restriction, and avoid the use of this agent for that reason.

NOTE: The absorption of penicillin-G from the G-I tract is variable; thus oral penicillin-G should not be used for severe infections.

Dosage: 250-500 mg every six (6) hours. *X 500mg q4h. BEST for 4 days.*

Parenteral route (injectable)/Aqueous Penicillin-G

Penicillin-G is an extremely valuable agent when administered parenterally. An example of an injectable form of the drug is crystalline penicillin-G sodium (also referred to as aqueous penicillin-G). It is indicated in the treatment of severe infections caused by penicillin-G-sensitive microorganisms when rapid and high penicillinemia is required. It is also indicated for prophylaxis against infectious endocarditis (see page 38). Aqueous penicillin-G is rapidly absorbed following intramuscular injection. Approximately 60% of the total dose is excreted in the urine within five hours. Therefore, high and frequent doses are required to maintain the elevated serum levels desirable in treating severe infections.

The **dosage range** is from 300,000 units to 4 million units every 6 hours. Since several injections daily are required, this agent has little practical use in dentistry except for obtaining an initial rapid blood level of penicillin which would be maintained with another dosage form such as oral penicillin-V or procaine penicillin-G by injection.

☐ Procaine Penicillin-G

Procaine penicillin-G dissolves slowly at the site of injection, giving a plateau type of blood level at about four hours, which falls slowly during the next 15 to 20 hours. It can be considered effective for 24 hours.

Dosage is 600,000 to 1,200,000 units once or twice daily. Procaine penicillin-G is also used for infectious endocarditis prophylaxis (see page 38).

☐ **Penicillin-V**

Penicillin-V is acid-stable and is dependably absorbed from the G-I tract. It resembles penicillin-G in its antibacterial action. On the basis of clinical effectiveness, it should rank as first choice among the oral penicillins.

The drug is administered as the free acid (penicillin-V) or as its potassium salt (penicillin V-K). The usual **dosage** is 250 to 500 mg every six (6) hours.

NOTE: The 500 mg dose is above that commonly recommended in your references. Penicillin is safe (for the non-allergic patient) up to levels as high as 2000 mg q.i.d. At these increased doses you achieve effectiveness against many oral anaerobic organisms (i.e., bacteroides species) which are resistant at the usual dosage (250 mg).

☐ **Dicloxacillin (or Cloxacillin)**

Dicloxacillin resists destruction by the enzyme penicillinase. It is not indicated in the treatment of routine oral infections and should be used only when a culture and sensitivity show it to be most effective **in vitro.** It is especially useful in the treatment of penicillinase-producing bacterial infections.

Dosage is 125 to 250 mg every six (6) hours.

☐ **Ampicillin**

Ampicillin is a synthetic penicillin with a broad spectrum of bacteriocidal activity against both penicillin susceptible gram-positive organisms and many common gram-negative pathogens. It has a special place as a standby antibiotic for dental purposes and should be reserved for infections with gram-negative organisms where bacterial susceptibility tests show it to be the preferred antibiotic. In fact, **it is rarely indicated in the treatment of dental infections.**

Dosage: 500 mg every six (6) hours.

Adverse reactions and principal drug interactions with penicillin

The principal adverse reaction is allergy (hypersensitivity). One should be alert to such symptoms as hives, itching, rash, or wheezing. There are no significant interactions with other drugs.

Allergic reactions to penicillins

Penicillins should not be prescribed for patients with either a past allergic reaction to penicillin or for patients with a history of allergies.

When prescribing penicillins you may wish to advise your patient of possible allergic reactions such as:

- hives
- itching
- rash
- respiratory difficulty

and advise them to:

- call you if they suspect any adverse side reaction
- call an ambulance or emergency aid car immediately if respiratory difficulty occurs

STUDY EXERCISE

1. PENICILLINS are the most useful and frequently prescribed antibiotics in dental use today.

2. If you have no culture and sensitivity data, what is the drug of choice as the "front line of treatment" for a dental infection? PENICILLIN

3. DICLOXACILLIN (CLOXACILLIN) is a penicillin resistant to destruction by penicillinase.

4. What is the principal adverse reaction to penicillin? ALLERGY
Describe its signs and symptoms. HIVES, ITCHING, RASH, WHEEZING

5. Which of the following can be given either orally or parenterally?
   a. Penicillin-V
   b. Penicillin-G (circled)
   c. Penicillin-B

6. If you receive a laboratory report on a bacterial culture stating that the infective organisms produce penicillinase, which of the following would you prescribe?
   a. Penicillin-V
   b. Penicillin-G
   c. Ampicillin
   d. Cloxacillin (circled)

ANSWERS

1. The penicillins
2. Penicillin
3. Dicloxacillin (or cloxacillin)
4. Allergy, hives, itching, rash or wheezing
5. b. Penicillin-G
6. d. Cloxacillin

• Erythromycin

This group of antibiotics is primarily effective against gram-positive organisms with a spectrum similar to penicillin. Its use in dentistry has been generally limited to individuals with a known hypersensitivity (allergy) to penicillin. Erythromycin stearate should be substituted for penicillin only when this is the case or when a specific microorganism has been shown to be sensitive to erythromycin and not to penicillin. Its oral absorption, like penicillin-G, is affected by gastric acidity. It is best administered on an empty stomach.

A more stable form, erythromycin estolate, has been developed which results in higher blood concentrations, even with food in the stomach. A major problem with the estolate form of the drug is hepatotoxicity which is reversible with discontinuation of the drug. **The estolate form will be withdrawn from the U.S. market because of its hepatotoxicity.** (FDA Drug Bulletin, Nov. 1979.)

Other side effects of the drug are relatively minor and usually include G-I upset, especially when the drug is given on an empty stomach. Allergic reactions are very rare.

Dosage: 250 mg every six (6) hours.

STUDY EXERCISE

1. *Erythromycin is primarily effective against gram* POSITIVE *organisms.*
2. *Erythromycin is the drug of choice when*
   a. *an individual is* ALLERGIC *to* PENICILLIN.
   b. *sensitivity tests show that the organism is* SENSITIVE *to erythromycin and* NOT SENSITIVE TO ~~*not*~~ *penicillin.*
3. *Should you tell your patients to take erythromycin before or after eating?* ______
   Why? 1 H BEFORE 2 H AFTER BECAUSE IT IS BROKEN DOWN BY ↓ STOMACH pH.
4. *Erythromycin* ESTOLATE *is stable in gastric acid, but will be withdrawn from the market because of its* HEPATOTOXICITY.

- **Tetracyclines**

All of the tetracyclines are very similar in their antimicrobial spectrum, their oral absorption, and in their side effects. They are bacteriostatic and inhibit a wide range of both gram-positive and gram-negative bacteria. There have been recent reports of tetracycline-resistant strains of Group A betahemolytic streptococci.

NOTE: Tetracyclines are not indicated in the treatment of any dental infection unless a microorganism sensitive to these drugs has been specifically found.

Side effects of tetracyclines include:

- Staining of teeth during amelogenesis
- Complaints of G-I upset (flatulence, nausea, vomiting, and diarrhea are fairly common)
- Rarely allergic reactions
- Toxic effects from this drug are rarely serious

Drug Interactions

Tetracycline should not be administered with any divalent-containing substance such as milk or antacid medications. The cations (such as calcium) combine with the tetracycline in the stomach and prevent absorption. The following are common drugs or compounds which can interact with the tetracyclines:

- aluminum, calcium, or magnesium-containing antacids
- iron supplements
- magnesium-containing laxatives

Dosage: 250 to 500 mg every six (6) hours

NOTE: Tetracycline should be taken with a full glass of water on an empty stomach (or with a little food if gastrointestinal irritation is a problem) either one hour before or two hours after meals to obtain optimum blood levels.

STUDY EXERCISE

1. Tetracyclines are effective against gram POSITIVE AND NEGATIVE *organisms.*

2. What should you caution your patients about when taking tetracyclines?

a. Do not take them with DIVALENT *containing substances such as* MILK *or* ANTACIDS *.*

b. Take them with a(n) (empty/full) ____ *stomach.*

3. What side effect do tetracycline antibiotics have on developing teeth? STAINING DURING AMELOGENESES

- **Clindamycin and Lincomycin**

These two antibiotics have spectrums very similar to erythromycin (primarily gram-positive) and are considered by some to be acceptable substitutes for penicillin-hypersensitive patients and for patients with infections due to penicillinase-producing staphylococci. The primary use of lincomycin in dentistry has been for the treatment of osteomyelitis. It has been rarely used in oral infections unless the bacteria have shown to be sensitive to the drug.

Clindamycin (Cleocin) has a similar spectrum to lincomycin. It is more completely absorbed from the G-I tract. It should be used in oral infections only when specifically indicated by bacterial susceptibility testing. Clindamycin has been found to be especially effective against **bacteroides** infections which have been increasingly reported in the head and neck.

Side effects: The primary side effects of clindamycin and lincomycin are G-I upset and diarrhea. **Recent reports on clindamycin and lincomycin state that these drugs have been associated with instances of severe colitis, which may terminate in death.** Allergic reactions to either drug appear to be rare.

NOTE: It is strongly recommended that the use of clindamycin and lincomycin be strictly limited to those situations where susceptibility tests indicate these antibiotics to be the only drug of choice.

Drug Interactions

General anesthetics
Neuromuscular blocking agents
Antiperistoltic, antidiarrheals
Kaolin-containing antidiarrheals

Dosage: Clindamycin — 150 to 450 mg every six (6) hours
Lincomycin — 500 mg every six to eight hours

STUDY EXERCISE

1. *Clindamycin and lincomycin are primarily effective against gram* POSITIVE *organisms.*

2. *The primary use of lincomycin in dentistry has been for* OSTEOMYELITIS *.*

3. CLINDAMYCIN *has been found to be effective against bacteroides infections of the head and neck.*

4. *Both clindamycin and lincomycin cause* G-I UPSET *as a side effect.*

5. CLINDAMYCIN *should be used only when found to be the drug of choice because it has been associated with severe* COLITIS *which may be fatal.*

• Cephalosporins

Two representatives of this family of antibiotics are available for oral administration. They are **cephalexin** and **cephalorodine.** They are similar agents and can be used almost interchangeably. For reasons of space, only cephalexin will be described here.

Cephalexin is a semi-synthetic cephalosporin intended for oral administration. It is acid stable and may be given without regard to meals. It is rapidly absorbed.

It is bacteriocidal against a broad spectrum of strep and staph organisms. However, its use in anaerobic infections is not approved by the United States Food and Drug Administration (FDA)[1]. Cephalexin is most frequently indicated for respiratory tract and urinary tract infections.

In dentistry it should be used only when specifically indicated by a susceptibility test or in some cases when the patient is allergic to penicillin. Cephalexin should not be regarded as a first choice antibiotic. It should be considered a reserve antibiotic.

Dosage: Up to 4 gm daily. Usual dosage is 250 mg every six (6) hours

Adverse reactions:

- allergic reactions
- diarrhea

STUDY EXERCISES

1. *Cephalosporins are effective against a broad spectrum of* STREP *and* STAPH *organisms.*

2. *What will you tell your patients about taking cephalosporins before, after or during meals?* NO REGARD TO MEALS

3. *Cephalosporin should be considered a* RESERVE *antibiotic and prescribed when* INDICATED BY A SUSCEPTIBILITY TEST OR PENICILLIN ALLERGY *.*

[1]American Medical Association. AMA Drug Evaluations, 3rd ed. Acton, Mass. Publishing Sciences Group, Inc. 1977.

Aminoglycosides

The aminoglycosides are used almost exclusively to treat gram-negative infections. The most commonly used aminoglycosides are streptomycin, kanamycin and gentamycin. They are all given either IM or IV.

NOTE: These antibiotics are both nephrotoxic and ototoxic, and their non-specific use is unwise.

STUDY EXERCISE

1. *Aminoglycosides are effective against gram* NEGATIVE *organisms.*

2. *Non-specific use of aminoglycosides is* UNWISE *because they are* NEPHROTOXIC *and* OTOTOXIC.

3. *Three commonly used aminoglycosides are* STREPTOMYCIN, KANAMYCIN *and* GENTAMYCIN.

REVIEW EXERCISES

From the following ***list of penicillins,*** *select which drug would be the best to use and write out a prescription and regimen for the antibiotic of choice for the following clinical situations.*

A. Penicillin-G
B. Penicillin-V
C. Procaine penicillin-G
D. Ampicillin
E. Sodium Dicloxacillin

1. *A 19-year-old patient appears with acute cellulitis of the right canine fossa. His past medical history reveals no allergies.*

   Drug: PEN-V 500 mg
   Disp: 28 TABS
   Sig: 1 TAB QID

2. *A 17-year-old female, following the removal of third molars, appears at your office with acute infection of the submandibular space. This is the fifth post-operative day and the patient had already had an incision and drainage on the third post-operative day. At that time she was placed on penicillin-V but without response. The bacteriologic report indicates that the organisms are penicillinase-producing staphylococci.*

   Drug: Na^+-DICLOXACILLIN 250 mg
   Disp: 28 CAPS
   Sig: 2 CAPS q6h

3. A 10-year-old male (weight 75 lbs.) reports to your office with an acute infection about the mandibular right deciduous molar. Past medical history reveals no allergies. An incision and drainage of the area was performed and you note that the Gram stain reveals both Gram-positive cocci and a significant number of Gram-negative rods.

Drug: AMPICILLIN 125 mg
Disp: 28 CAPS
Sig: 1 CAP q 6 h

For questions 4-7, **choose from the non-penicillin antibiotics** and complete the inscription, subscription and signatura you would use on the prescription.

4. A patient presents with a severe pericoronitis. You exude some pus and determine the organism is Gram-positive. The patient is allergic to penicillin.

Inscription	Subscription	Signatura
ERYTHROMYCIN STEARATE 500 mg	28 TABS	1 TAB q 6 h

5. A 20-year-old female with an infection secondary to the removal of third molars reports to your office. The patient had been placed on penicillin on the third day post-operatively, at which time an incision and drainage had been attempted. This is the fifth post-operative day and there has been no improvement. The culture shows sensitivity to cephalothin.

Inscription	Subscription	Signatura
CEPHALEXIN 250 mg	28 TABS	1 TAB q 6 h

6. A 54-year-old male with a history of a fractured mandible 8 weeks ago appears at your office with a swelling of the left mandibular angle that has been present for about one and a half weeks. Despite adequate penicillin therapy, a radiograph reveals that the swelling is in the area of the old fracture and that there is a radiolucency consistent with osteomyelitis. This, in fact, is the diagnosis. What antibiotic would you prescribe for him?

Inscription	Subscription	Signatura
CLINDAMYCIN 300 mg	28 TABS	1 TAB q 6 h

ANSWERS TO REVIEW EXERCISES

Case #1
Drug: Penicillin-V 500 mg
Disp: 28 tablets
Sig: 1 tablet qid

Case #2
Drug: Sodium Dicloxacillin 250 mg
Disp: 28 capsules
Sig: 2 capsules every 6 hours

Case #3
Drug: Ampicillin 125 mg
Disp: 28 capsules
Sig: 1 capsule every 6 hours

Case #4
Drug: Erythromycin Stearate 500 mg
Disp: 28 tablets
Sig: 1 tablet q 6 hr

Case #5
Drug: Cephalexin 250 mg
Disp: 28 tablets
Sig: 1 tablet q 6 hr

Case #6
Drug: Clindamycin 300 mg
Disp: 28 tablets
Sig: 1 tablet q 6 hr

PROPHYLACTIC USE OF ANTIBIOTICS

Antibiotics should not be used prophylactically except for specific indications.

Principle Prophylactic Indications for Antibiotic Therapy

1. History of acquired rheumatic or other valvular heart disease.
2. Prosthetic heart valves.
3. Congenital heart disease.
4. Recent steroid therapy.
5. Anti-neoplastic chemotherapy.
6. Implants used in orthopedic surgery (e.g., silastic or metallic joints).
7. Any disease which limits the patient's ability to respond to infections

American Heart Association Dosage Guidelines for Prophylaxis (1977) for patients with a history of rheumatic or other acquired heart disease and most congenital heart diseases

Parenteral-Oral Combined

Adults
Aqueous crystalline penicillin-G (1,000,000 units IM) mixed with procaine penicillin-G (600,000 units IM). Give 30 minutes to 1 hour prior to procedure, and then give penicillin-V 500 mg orally every six hours for eight doses.

Children
Aqueous crystalline penicillin-G (30,000 units/Kg. IM) mixed with procaine penicillin-G (600,000 units IM). Timing of doses is the same as for adults. For children less than 60 pounds, the dose of penicillin-V is 250 mg orally every six hours for eight doses.

Oral

Adults
Penicillin-V (2.0 gm orally) 30 minutes to 1 hour prior to the procedure, and then 500 mg orally every 6 hours for 8 doses.

Children
Penicillin-V (2.0 gm orally) 30 minutes to 1 hour prior to procedure, and then 500 mg orally every 6 hours for 8 doses. For children less than 60 pounds, use 1.0 gm orally 30 minutes to 1 hour prior to the procedure, and then 250 mg orally every 6 hours for 8 doses.

Patients Allergic to Penicillin

Adults
Erythromycin (1.0 gm orally) 1½ - 2 hours prior to the procedure, and then 500 mg orally every 6 hours for 8 doses.

Children
Erythromycin (1.0 gm orally) 1½ - 2 hours prior to the procedure, and then 10 mg/Kg every 6 hours for 8 doses.

Patients with Prosthetic Heart Valves

Penicillin plus streptomycin

Adults

Aqueous crystalline penicillin-G (1,000,000 units IM) mixed with procaine penicillin-G (600,000 units IM) plus streptomycin (1 gm IM). Give 30 minutes to 1 hour prior to the procedure, then penicillin-V 500 mg orally every 6 hours for 8 doses.

Children

Aqueous crystalline penicillin-G (30,000 units/Kg IM) mixed with procaine penicillin-G (600,000 units IM), plus streptomycin (20 mg/Kg IM). Timing of doses for children is same as for adults. For children less than 60 pounds, the recommended oral dose of penicillin is 250 mg every 6 hours for 8 doses.

Patients Allergic to Penicillin

Adults

Vancomycin (1 gm IV over 30 minutes to 1 hour). Start initial vancomycin infusion ½ to 1 hour prior to procedure, then erythromycin 500 mg orally every 6 hours for 8 doses.

Children

Vancomycin (20 mg/Kg IV over 30 minutes to 1 hour). Timing of doses for children is the same as for adults. Erythromycin dose is 10 mg/Kg every 6 hours for 8 doses.

Before initiating antibiotic prophylaxis, you should always consult with the patient's physician. It should be emphasized that this consultation is only for advice and that you are primarily responsible for this part of the treatment of the patient. If the physician suggests a smaller dose of antibiotics, you have the option of following this advice or the guidelines provided by the AHA. If the physician advises more aggressive therapy, you should follow the suggestion. The use of antibiotics other than penicillin and erythromycin should be discouraged unless the patient is allergic to both. In this case, consult with an internist or cardiologist for an acceptable substitute.

TO RE-EMPHASIZE, YOU SHOULD NOT USE ANTIBIOTICS PROPHYLACTICALLY FOR ANY BUT THE ABOVE REASONS, EXCEPT WHERE IT CAN BE DEMONSTRATED THAT IT WILL BE OF BENEFIT TO THE PATIENT.

STUDY EXERCISE

1. *The recommended drug for antibiotic prophylaxis for patients with rheumatic heart disease, acquired heart disease and congenital heart disease is* PENICILLIN *.* *If the patient is allergic to this then you should substitute* ERYTHROMYCIN *.*
2. *Antibiotic prophylaxis is indicated any time you are concerned about post-operative infection. True or false?* ____
3. *State five indications for prophylactic antibiotic therapy.*
   a. RHD
   b. PROSTH. HEART VALVES
   c. CONGENITAL HEART DISEASE
   d. STEROID THERAPY
   e. CHEMOTHERAPY IMPLANTS
4. *Penicillin plus streptomycin is recommended for antibiotic prophylaxis for patients with* PROSTHETIC HEART VALVES *.*

ANTIBIOTICS AND THEIR USUAL ADULT DOSAGES

- Penicillin-G (page 29)
  250 - 500 mg
  every 4 hours
- Penicillin-V (page 30)
  250 - 500 mg
  every 6 hours
- Procaine Penicillin (page 29)
  600,000 - 1,200,000 units
  once or twice daily
- Dicloxacillin (page 30)
  125 - 250 mg
  every 6 hours
- Ampicillin (page 30)
  250 - 500 mg
  every 6 hours
- Tetracyclines (page 33)
  Dosage differs among the varieties
- Erythromycin Stearate (page 32)
  250 mg
  every 6 hours
- Lincomycin (page 34)
  500 mg
  every 6 hours
- Clindamycin (page 34)
  150 - 300 mg
  every 6 hours
- Cephalexin (page 35)
  250 - 500 mg
  every 6 hours

NOTE: Do not attempt to memorize these dosages. Be sure to reconfirm each dosage when you are writing the prescription.

Unit IV

ANALGESICS

Mild Analgesics
- **Aspirin**
- **Ibuprofen**
- **Acetaminophen**
- **Propoxyphene**

Moderate Analgesics
- **Codeine plus Aspirin**
- **Codeine plus Acetaminophen**

Strong Analgesics
- **Meperidine**
- **Pentazocine**
- **Oxycodone**

Guidelines for Analgesic Use in Oral Surgery

PRETEST

- Answer the following questions.
- Compare your responses with the correct responses given.
- If all responses were correct, you have finished this chapter.
- If only some responses were correct, proceed to Unit IV, page 44.
- The numbers in parentheses refer to the specific objective number from which the questions were derived.

QUESTIONS

1. *Rank the following analgesics as to their relative potency, from mildest to strongest (03-04-04).*

	Mild	Moderate	Strong
a. Acetaminophen			
b. Propoxyphene hydrochloride			
c. Meperidine			
d. Pentazocine			
e. Oxycodone			
f. Ibuprofen			
g. Codeine 30 mg plus Aspirin 325 mg			

2. *Describe how analgesics can be combined to provide a greater amount of pain relief for the patient (03-04-05).* __________

3. *Which of the following drugs are narcotics with potential for abuse and/or addiction (03-04-03)?*
   - a. Acetaminophen
   - b. Demerol
   - c. Propoxyphene
   - d. Codeine
   - e. Oxycodone
   - f. Meperidine
   - g. Aspirin
   - h. Pentazocine

4. *Two adverse effects of aspirin are a)* __________ *and b) decreased* __________ *(03-04-03).*

5. *An overdose of acetaminophen may cause* __________ *and/or* __________ *(03-04-03).*

6. A major cause of drug-related deaths is excessive doses of PROPOXYPHENE either alone or in combination with CNS depressants (03-04-03).

7. Pain medications are usually required for 1 - 2 days following oral surgery (03-04-01).

8. Describe the three groups of oral surgical procedures presented in this chapter which can be expected to result in differing levels of pain post-operatively (03-04-04).
   Group I UNCOMPLICATED SINGLE EXTRACTION
   Group II MUCOPERIOSTEAL FLAP.
   Group III MUCOPERIOSTEAL FLAP + BONE REMOVAL.

9. Whatever drug you prescribe for post-operative pain, it is important that you take full advantage of its PLACEBO effect (03-04-01)

10. Give a clinical example of when to use the following drugs (03-04-04):
    a. Aspirin 650 mg. UNCOMPLICATE SINGLE EXTRACTION
    b. Propoxyphene napsylate 100 mg with acetaminophen 650 mg. UNCOMPLICATED EXTRACTION OR CODEINE INTOLERANCE.
    c. Codeine 30 mg with aspirin 650 mg. MOST EXTRACTIONS
    d. Meperidine 100 mg. DIFFICULT EXTRACTIONS.

11. IBUPROFEN is similar to aspirin in its anti-inflammatory, anti-pyretic and analgesic properties (03-04-02).

12. You planned to recommend aspirin to a patient for pain relief, but find that he is allergic to it. What are two non-narcotic substitutes you could suggest (03-04-02)?
    a. ACETAMINOPHEN
    b. IBUPROFEN

ANSWERS

1. a. mild
   b. mild
   c. strong
   d. strong
   e. strong
   f. mild
   g. moderate

2. Combine a narcotic (or narcotic-like drug) with aspirin or acetaminophen at their individual effective doses.

3. b, c, d, e, f, h

4. a. Gastro-intestinal bleeding
   b. Decreased platelet aggregation

5. Renal injury, death

6. Propoxyphene

7. 1 - 2

8. Group I — Uncomplicated single extraction
   Group II — Procedure utilizing a mucoperiosteal flap
   Group III — Procedure utilizing a mucoperiosteal flap and extensive bone removal

9. Placebo

10. Any answer similar to examples below. Might give examples such as:
    a. Uncomplicated single extraction
    b. Uncomplicated impaction or codeine intolerance
    c. Most impactions
    d. Difficult extractions

11. Ibuprofen

12. a. Acetaminophen
    b. Ibuprofen

Unit IV

ANALGESICS

Introduction
Mild Analgesics
- Aspirin
- Ibuprofen
- Acetaminophen
- Codeine
- Propoxyphene

Moderate Analgesics
- Codeine plus Aspirin
- Codeine plus Acetaminophen

Strong Analgesics
- Meperidine
- Pentazocine
- Oxycodone

Guidelines for analgesic use in oral surgery

INTRODUCTION

The treatment of pain is one of the prime functions of the dentist. It is especially important that you be familiar with the types of drugs necessary to relieve or control pain associated with oral surgical procedures.

Post-operative pain per se cannot be considered a complication of surgery. The experienced surgeon will recognize normal post-operative pain patterns. There are anatomic variables with regard to the pain response. For example, surgery performed on the maxilla is generally less painful than surgery on the mandible. Surgical procedures performed on the anterior portion of the mandible are usually less painful than those in the third molar region. These generalizations may prove useful in selecting the most appropriate analgesic for your patient.

Patient variables must also be kept in mind. At either end of the range of normal threshold levels for response to pain there is a group of patients who are either hypersensitive or hyposensitive to pain. The hypersensitive patient will appear to complain excessively over minor discomforts. Conversely, the hyposensitive patient will rarely require analgesics following dental procedures. It has been suggested by some that these traits of low or high pain tolerance are inborn characteristics. Others have suggested a cultural or even an ethnic relationship.

In the following description of the various analgesic agents, there is a reference to relative potency of these agents. This should be viewed in the same way as the EPA (United States Environmental Protection Agency) mileage ratings for automobiles. These ratings are not valid for an individual automobile, but they are regarded as valid in comparing one type of car to another type. Because of individual patient variables, each patient will respond differently to a given analgesic.

The placebo effect must also be considered and in certain instances exploited. The power of suggestion should not be underestimated. Recent research related to the placebo effect has suggested that the brain is capable of secreting its own narcotic called endorphin. This fascinating research finally offers an explanation for the long-recognized placebo effect.

The enthusiasm of the prescriber has been shown to increase the proportion of patients obtaining relief by medication from any type of pain. The analgesic effect of a drug may also be increased by dispensing it as a brightly-colored capsule or tablet, once again exploiting the possible placebo effect.

In the majority of cases, severe pain is not typical following oral surgical procedures, and the choice of analgesic agents is not critical.

When you are especially concerned about the efficacy of an analgesic agent, you should prescribe the maximum therapeutic amount of the drug. For example, the most common analgesic medications such as codeine with aspirin or acetaminophen are usually prescribed at half or less of the maximum therapeutic amount (codeine 30 mg with aspirin 325 mg). When moderate to extreme pain is expected, the full therapeutic amount should be given, i.e., codeine 30 to 60 mg with aspirin 650 mg or acetaminophen 1000 mg.

Analgesic drugs are frequently mixed to take advantage of an additive effect. For example, a narcotic such as codeine is commonly mixed with aspirin because the codeine acts on the central nervous system while aspirin acts at the site of injury. In most instances it is wise to take advantage of this additive effect.

STRATEGY FOR POST-OPERATIVE ANALGESIA

There is an extremely variable amount of pain during the first eight hours following surgery. The pain can be very severe. A definite strategy with regard to the control of post-operative pain is useful in tiding the patient over this difficult period. It is hard to "catch up" on pain medication if the patient reports extreme pain in the immediate post-operative period without adequate analgesic relief.

An example of strategy for pain relief following the removal of a mandibular third molar would be as shown in **Figure IV-1**. During the first twelve hours (first three doses), your patient should take the oxycodone plus **two** 500 mg acetaminophen tablets; during the next eighteen hours (second three doses) take oxycodone plus **one** 500 mg acetaminophen tablet; and then during the following eighteen hours (next three doses) discontinue oxycodone but increase acetaminophen back to **two** 500 mg tablets. This strategy is suggested only for those extremely difficult extractions where acute pain is anticipated.

NOTE: Following difficult extractions, patients take analgesics for an average of two days.

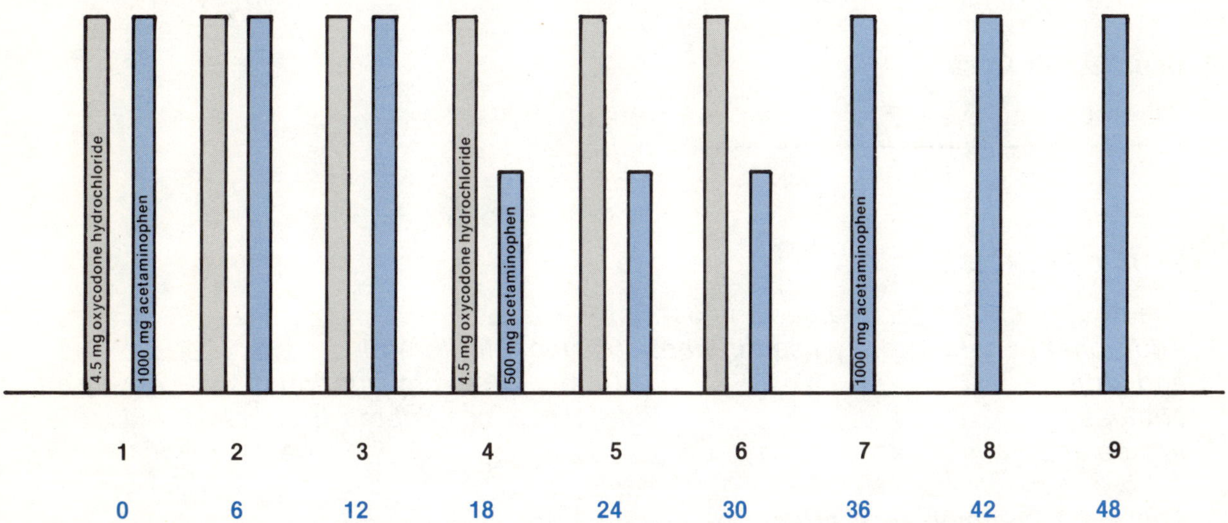

Figure IV-1. Timing strategies for prescribing oxycodone hydrochloride in combination with acetaminophen to ensure maximum analgesic effect during the most painful post-operative time period. Black numbers under figure represent dose number; blue numbers represent post-surgical time in hours.

MILD ANALGESICS

• Aspirin

This agent is the drug of choice when a mild analgesic is indicated. Aspirin has the additional benefit of being anti-inflammatory and antipyretic, although these effects are rarely used in dentistry. When deciding on a mild analgesic, aspirin should always receive prime consideration. An alternative is used only when there is a decided advantage to the other drug, either in improved analgesia or in a decrease of side effects. Aspirin has been shown to inhibit the synthesis of prostaglandins which are thought to cause pain, inflammation, and edema at the traumatized site.

Adverse Reactions

Serious adverse reactions with usual analgesic doses occur infrequently. Gastrointestinal symptoms such as dyspepsia, nausea, and vomiting are most common. Occult gastrointestinal bleeding occurs in many patients but is usually clinically insignificant. Because usual doses of aspirin inhibit platelet aggregation, thereby affecting coagulation, the drug is contraindicated in patients with bleeding disorders.

Some clinicians who prefer to use aspirin for its anti-inflammatory effects will use acetaminophen 24 hours following surgery because of aspirin's ability to inhibit platelet aggregation. Other clinicians feel this to be unnecessary.

A small percentage of individuals are hypersensitive to aspirin. Even usual doses may cause rash or severe urticarial or asthmatic type of anaphylactic reactions in these patients. The incidence of sensitivity is higher in patients with asthma, hay fever or nasal polyps.

Drug Interactions

- other anti-inflammatory medications
- anticoagulants
- oral hypoglycemics (effects of these medications may be increased when used concurrently with aspirin)
- methotrexate

Usual Adult Dose

325 to 650 mg every 3 to 4 hours as needed.

STUDY EXERCISE

The drug of choice for analgesia in dentistry is ____________________. Additional benefits, rarely used in dentistry, include its anti-____________________ and anti-____________________ effects. When considering the use of any mild analgesic ____________________ should be considered first unless a decrease in side effects is necessary or a more ____________________ analgesic is needed.

The most common side effects of aspirin involve ____________________-symptoms. It should not be prescribed for patients with ulcers because it causes ____________________ ____________________. Patients with bleeding disorders should not take aspirin because it causes decreased ____________________.

- **Ibuprofen (Motrin)**

Ibuprofen is one of a new series of phenylalkanoic acid derivates that has been recently marketed as an antiarthritic agent. Its analgesic, anti-inflammatory and anti-pyretic properties resemble aspirin. Cooper, et al.[1] have demonstrated that ibuprofen is not only more potent as an analgesic than aspirin, but has greater efficacy without any notable increase in adverse effects. Thus, it may be used as an aspirin substitute or when a slightly more potent analgesic agent is required.

Adverse Reactions

Patients hypersensitive to aspirin or other non-steroidal anti-inflammatories may be hypersensitive to this medication also.

Drug Interactions

Alcohol
Other anti-inflammatory agents
Anti-coagulants

Usual Adult Dose

400 - 600 mg every four hours as needed (up to 2.4 grams daily)

NOTE: The true analgesic and anti-inflammatory value of the phenylalkanoic acid derivatives (such as ibuprofen and fenbufen) in the treatment of dental pain has not as yet emerged in the scientific literature due to the relatively short time this group of drugs has been marketed. Because of the recent significance of this drug group, we have included at the end of this chapter a listing of published papers on their use in dentistry. All indications thus far are that this group is a bright star on the horizon. However, you should follow the literature over the next few years.

STUDY EXERCISES

Ibuprofen is similar to aspirin in its ANTI-INFLAMMATORY, ANTIPYRETIC *and* ANALGESIC *properties.*

(Ibuprofen/Aspirin) ______________________ *is more potent than (ibuprofen/aspirin)* ______________________ *.*

Ibuprofen (would/would not) ______________________ *be a good substitute for aspirin if your patient is allergic to aspirin.*

---

[1]Cooper, S.A., Needle, S.E., Kruger, G.O., Comparative Analgesic Potency of Aspirin and Ibuprofen, J. Oral Surgery, vol. 35, November, 1977.

- **Acetaminophen**

As an analgesic, acetaminophen is equal to aspirin. However, it lacks aspirin's anti-inflammatory effect. Acetaminophen does not cause gastrointestinal bleeding or affect platelet aggregation as does aspirin. It is probably the analgesic of choice as an alternative to aspirin, particularly in patients allergic to aspirin or with a history of peptic ulcer.

Adverse Reactions

Prolonged use of acetaminophen may cause renal injury. Hepatic necrosis and death have been observed following overdosage. Hepatic damage is likely if an adult has taken a single dose of more than 10 grams or if a three-year-old child has taken more than 3 grams.

Drug Interaction

Large doses have been reported to potentiate the action of oral anticoagulants.

Usual Adult Dose

One to four 325 mg tablets (325 - 1300 mg) every four hours as neded. Available in 325 and 500 mg tablets or capsules.

In the Hopkinson study[1], it has been shown that 1,300 mg of acetaminophen produces significantly greater analgesia than does 650 mg. Therefore, when prescribing acetaminophen, inform your patient that doubling the usual dose (650 mg) is safe for a short period of time and will be more effective in reducing pain if the lower dose has not been sufficient.

STUDY EXERCISE

Acetaminophen is as effective an analgesic as aspirin. However, it lacks aspirin's ANTI-INFLAMMATORY *effect.*

Acetaminophen does not cause GI *bleeding or affect* PLATELET *aggregation. Prolonged use, however, will cause* RENAL *injury.*

HEPATIC *damage and death have been observed following overdosage.*

If a patient's pain is not relieved by 650 mg of acetaminophen, what would you recommend? DOUBLE THE DOSE.

[1]Hopkinson, J. H., et al.: Curr. Ther. Res. 16:194 (March) 1974.

• Codeine

Codeine is useful in relieving mild to moderate pain. Codeine contributes to analgesia by a mechanism not fully known, although there is evidence to indicate that narcotic analgesics act on opiate receptors in the brain. While aspirin seems to act peripherally, codeine and other narcotics act on the central nervous system. An oral dose of 30 mg of codeine is approximately equivalent to 650 mg of aspirin. 15 mg of codeine is usually ineffective. Codeine has been reported to be less effective than aspirin (when used alone) in managing dental pain. For this reason, it is ordinarily used in combination with another analgesic for managing post-operative pain.

Adverse Reactions

The most common reactions are nausea, vomiting, sedation, and dizziness. **Your patient should be advised not to drive whenever taking prescribed narcotics such as codeine.**

Drug Interactions

Drug interactions with narcotics can be serious. Drugs interacting with narcotics include:

alcohol
CNS depressants
monoamine oxidase inhibitors
tricyclic antidepressants

Usual Adult Dose

The usual dose of codeine is 30 mg. An increased analgesic effect is produced with larger doses (60 mg) but the incidence of undesirable side effects is increased. These doses are recommended every four hours as needed.

NOTE: Codeine, when prescribed alone, is a Schedule II drug under the Controlled Substances Act. This means that there are specific limitations on its use, especially pertaining to the refilling of the prescription. **In most states, telephone orders are not permitted for Schedule II medications.**

• Codeine Cogeners

Hydrocodone and dihydrocodeine are two codeine cogeners which are approximately as effective as codeine with possibly slight advantages over codeine such as a slightly lower incidence of nausea and vomiting.

Usual Adult Dose

Hydrocodone 5 mg and acetaminophen 500 mg every four hours.
Dihydrocodeine 16 mg, promethazine 6.25 mg with APC

STUDY EXERCISE

Codeine is useful in relieving ____________ to ____________ pain. It has been reported to be (more/less) ____________ effective than aspirin when used alone.

Prescribing doses greater or less than 30 mg of codeine on a routine basis (may/may not) ____________ be effective therapy.

Side effects of codeine are those of narcotics; in general, they include: (1) ____________ (2) ____________, (3) ____________, and (4) ____________.

When prescribed alone, codeine is a Schedule ____________ drug. Telephone orders (are/are not) ____________ permitted in most states.

- **Propoxyphene Hydrochloride and Napsylate**

Propoxyphene is a mild narcotic analgesic closely related to methadone in chemical structure, and thus should be considered in the class of weak narcotics. There is a widespread debate as to the relative value of propoxyphene over aspirin in treatment of mild pain. The consensus is that propoxyphene is no more effective and usually is less so than 650 mg of aspirin. Propoxyphene does not provide any anti-inflammatory action.

Adverse Reactions

Abuse of propoxyphene with the development of morphine-type dependence has been reported; however, its dependence liability is less than with codeine. Nevertheless, because propoxyphene may be abused by some patients and death may result from overdosage, you should use caution in prescribing this drug.

NOTE: Propoxyphene products in excessive doses, either alone or in combination with other central nervous system depressants, including alcohol, are a major cause of drug-related deaths.

The following warnings apply to the use of propoxyphene compounds:

1. Do not prescribe propoxyphene for patients who are suicidal or addiction-prone.
2. Prescribe propoxyphene with caution for patients taking tranquilizers or antidepressant drugs and in patients who use alcohol in excess.
3. Tell your patients not to exceed the recommended dose and to limit their intake of alcohol.

Drug Interactions

alcohol
CNS depressants
MAO inhibitors
tricyclic antidepressants

Usual Adult Dose

One tablet or capsule every four hours as needed for any of the following preparations:

1. 65 mg of propoxyphene hydrochloride
2. 100 mg of propoxyphene napsylate
3. 65 mg of propoxyphene hydrochloride and 325 mg of aspirin
4. 65 mg of propoxyphene hydrochloride with APC
5. 65 mg of propoxyphene hydrochloride and either 325 or 650 mg of acetaminophen
6. 100 mg of propoxyphene napsylate and 650 mg of acetaminophen

NOTE: Because of patient abuse potential for propoxyphene compounds and the seriousness of potential drug interactions, you would be wise to avoid the use of propoxyphene for treatment of dental pain if other drugs can be used.

STUDY EXERCISE

Propoxyphene is a (strong/mild) ______ analgesic closely related to methadone and can be considered a weak ______.

Propoxyphene is believed to be less effective than ______ mg of ______ and (does/does not) ______ provide anti-inflammatory action.

Adverse reactions to propoxyphene include (a) morphine-type ______ and (b) death due to ______ or combination with other ______ ______.

You should not prescribe propoxyphene for patients who are ______ and use caution when prescribing it for patients taking ______ or who drink alcoholic beverages.

MODERATE ANALGESICS

It has been found that combinations of narcotics or narcotic derivatives, such as codeine with aspirin or acetaminophen, provide greater levels of analgesia than either drug given separately. Additive effects probably occur because the drugs act at different sites in the body. Although very little is known about the actions of the drugs, it is commonly accepted that the narcotics act in the central nervous system (centrally acting), and aspirin and acetaminophen act locally at the site of trauma (peripherally acting). The two sites of action are used to explain the experimental findings that, to be effective, both drugs have to be given at their normally effective dose levels.

In dentistry, codeine is usually combined with aspirin or acetaminophen, both of which produce an additive analgesic effect which is useful for treating mild to moderate pain. The following numbering scheme is traditionally used in identifying the amount of codeine in the mixture:

#1. Codeine — 7.5 mg
#2. Codeine — 15 mg
#3. Codeine — 30 mg
#4. Codeine — 60 mg

- **Codeine Phosphate Tablets plus Aspirin**

Usual Adult Dose

30 mg of codeine phosphate and 325 mg of aspirin. Take one or two tablets every four hours as needed.

- **Codeine Phosphate plus Acetaminophen**

Usual Adult Dose

One tablet containing 325 mg of acetaminophen and 30 mg of codeine phosphate every four hours as needed or one tablet containing 650 mg of acetaminophen and 30 mg of codeine phosphate every four hours as needed.

NOTE: Since 1,000 mg of acetaminophen is the desired therapeutic dose, it may be necessary to supplement the prescribed drug with plain acetaminophen. For example, the patient may take 650 mg of acetaminophen and 30 mg of codeine with one additional tablet of 325 mg of acetaminophen.

NOTE: With all codeine combinations, the patient should be advised that the medication may cause drowsiness. Therefore driving is not permitted. The patient should further avoid alcoholic beverages. In order to decrease the incidence of nausea, the medication should be taken with food or milk.

NOTE: When codeine is combined with aspirin or acetaminophin, it is a Schedule III narcotic. Telephone orders are permitted in most states.

STUDY EXERCISE

The combination of analgesics that provides additional analgesic protection are those that contain both a NARCOTIC *and either* ASPIRIN *or* ACETAMINOPHEN
How is this explained? ACTS CENTRALLY / ACTS PERIPHERALLY
____
____

Another advantage of this is that you are able to REDUCE *the amount of each drug, thus minimizing* ADVERSE REACTIONS *of one and increasing the benefits of another.*

Often, optimum analgesia using a codeine and aspirin (or acetaminophen) combination requires that your patient take additional ACETAMINOPHEN OR ASPIRIN.

Is it legal for you to prescribe a codeine and acetaminophen compound over the telephone? YES

STRONG ANALGESICS

- **Meperidine (Demerol, Pethidine)**

Meperidine is a narcotic drug. Unquestionably it provides improved analgesia over aspirin or codeine, but with this increased effectiveness comes an increase in side effects. Meperidine can be used orally in doses of 50 to 100 mg. Dosages in excess of 150 mg can produce significant respiratory depression. It is more common to see other side effects such as nausea, vomiting, and drowsiness. Patients should always be warned not to operate a motor vehicle or any other mechanical equipment while taking this drug. The abuse liability of this drug is moderately high and has been well-documented. When a strong analgesic is needed, oxycodone may be a superior choice.

NOTE: When prescribing meperidine, dispense only enough for one day and then switch to a less potent drug thereafter.

Adverse Reactions

nausea
vomiting
dizziness
respiratory depression

Drug Interactions

alcohol
CNS depressants
tricyclic antidepressants
monoamine oxidase inhibitors

Usual Adult Dose

50 to 150 mg every three to four hours as needed for pain.

STUDY EXERCISE

Meperidine provides considerably more analgesia than ________ or ________ but has (increased/no increase) ________ effects. Doses of ________ to ________ mg are commonly used via oral route. ________ mg is usually all that is needed for most out-patient oral surgery. With doses above 150 mg respiratory ________ may be significant. Other narcotic side effects such as (1) ________, (2) ________, and (3) ________ are more common.

While on this drug patients (should/should not) ________ operate ________ or other mechanical ________.

Abuse liability is ________ and well documented, and in patients who are ________ drug users or ________ this drug should not be used.

- **Pentazocine (Talwin)**

Pentazocine is a weak narcotic antagonist. It is effective in relieving moderate pain. It has no anti-inflammatory activity. The analgesic potency is approximately equal to codeine.

Adverse Reactions

nausea
vomiting
dizziness

Drug Interactions

alcohol
CNS depressants
other narcotic drugs (may cause withdrawal symptoms)

Usual Adult Dose

50 mg every three to four hours. Dosage may be increased to 100 mg every 3 to 4 hours. The total daily dose must not exceed 600 mg.

Pentazocine is also available mixed with aspirin. The usual dose is 325 mg aspirin and 12.5 mg of pentazocine, 2 tablets, 3 or 4 times a day as needed.

NOTE: Pentazocine is frequently prescribed in those instances when the patient is allergic to other analgesics.

Pentazocine is also available mixed with aspirin. The usual dose is 325 mg aspirin and 12.5 mg of pentazocine, 2 tablets, 3 or 4 times a day as needed.

STUDY EXERCISE

Pentazocine hydrochloride or (TALWIN) is a weak narcotic ANTAGONIST. Recent evidence indicates this drug to be about as potent as CODEINE.

Adverse reactions to this drug include:
a) NAUSEA
b) VOMITING
c) DIZZINESS

Pentazocine hydrochloride is CONTRAINDICATED *in treatment of patients with drug dependence on narcotics, since it will produce* WITHDRAWAL *symptoms.*

- **Oxycodone**

Oxycodone is effective in the treatment of moderately severe pain. It has greater analgesic potency as well as more dependence liability than codeine.

Oxycodone is not available alone. It is mixed with either acetaminophen or aspirin.

While this drug is very useful in alleviating moderately severe pain, its frequent abuse causes problems for most dentists. It should never be prescribed routinely nor should it be prescribed for a suspected drug abuser.

Adverse Reactions

dependence
CNS depression
drowsiness
nausea or vomiting

Drug Interactions

alcohol
CNS depressants
MAO inhibitors
tricyclic antidepressants

Usual Adult Dose

Several compounded products are available including:

1. 5 mg oxycodone hydrochloride **plus** 325 acetaminophen **or** 650 mg aspirin every six hours as needed.

2. 4.5 mg oxycodone hydrochloride, 0.38 mg oxycodone trepthalate **plus** 500 mg acetaminophen **or** 600 mg aspirin every six hours as needed.

STUDY EXERCISE

Oxycodone is effective in treatment of ____________ pain. It has greater analgesic potency and ____________ liability than ____________.

Oxycodone is available alone or in combination with aspirin or acetaminophen. True or false? ________

Oxycodone should not be prescribed routinely because of the potential for ____________ ____________.

GUIDELINES FOR ANALGESIC USE IN ORAL SURGERY

The choice of which analgesic to use for a patient following a specific procedure can vary widely, but depends primarily on your preference. This preference should be based on well-controlled studies as well as clinical experience. The following section on groupings of analgesics is based on the best available data on relative effectiveness. Each group gives you enough of a choice of analgesics to follow a personal preference. It must always be remembered that the "placebo effect" is a definite factor in providing analgesia. Thus, you have to believe that the drug you are prescribing is adequate for pain relief and you must try to convince your patient. If a patient has had a bad experience with one of the drugs in the group, you can easily select another drug and provide the same level of analgesia.

NOTE: Usually prescribe only enough analgesic for two days. If pain persists, you should examine your patient before prescribing more.

Usually analgesics are taken every three to four hours. The number of tablets that would last for two days would be 12 to 16.

Here are guidelines for the preceding groupings relative to their use in oral surgery. Drugs in each group will usually provide sufficient analgesic effect for the procedures listed.

Group I — A single uncomplicated extraction (extraction without the use of a flap)

Group II — An uncomplicated impaction or other oral surgical procedure in which a larger periosteal flap is raised.

Group III — A major oral surgical procedure, including impaction surgery involving a large flap and extensive bone removal

Remember that these are only relative reference points. You may find that your patients need more or less analgesia than suggested here. Be sure to take advantage of the placebo effect with all medications. Let the patient know that you are prescribing **effective** pain medications which you believe will control their pain.

GROUPING OF ANALGESICS BY RELATIVE ANALGESIC EFFECTIVENESS

1. **Group I**

Aspirin (ASA)	650 mg
Acetaminophen	650 mg
Codeine	30 mg
Ibuprofen	500 mg

2. **Group II**

Codeine	30 mg	plus aspirin	650 mg
Codeine	30 mg	plus acetaminophen	650 mg
Pentazocine	25 mg	plus aspirin	650 mg
Hydrocodone	5 mg	plus acetaminophen	500 mg

3. **Group III**

Meperidine (oral)	100 mg
Oxycodone	See page 55 for dose

STUDY EXERCISE

You should prescribe enough pain medication to last 2 days.
This is because you must examine patient if pain persists.

When prescribing analgesics it is important to take advantage of the placebo effect to get optimum pain relief.

Although there is some overlap between groups, oral surgical procedures have been divided into three groups or levels of anticipated pain. These groups are only a relative reference point and may be modified for individual patients. For each group state the types of procedures that might be expected to produce this level of pain:

Group I uncomplicated extraction
Group II uncomplicated impaction & flap
Group III major oral surgery, large flap, bone removal, impaction

For groups I and II name the two (2) analgesics you would like to use for treating that level of anticipated pain.

Group I (a) Aspirin
(b) Codeine
Group II (a) Aspirin & Codeine
(b) Acetaminophen & Codeine

For each of the following cases, state the inscription, subscription, and signatura for the analgesic of choice.

1. You have just removed a periodontally involved central incisor that has about a Class III mobility from a 55-year-old male. The patient claims he never takes any aspirin for headaches and generally does not like to take pills.
   a. Inscription Acetaminophen 650 mg.
   b. Subscription Disp: 32 tabs
   c. Signatura 2 tab each 3-4 hr's

2. An 18-year-old girl has two distoangular, Class 11B (difficult) impactions removed in the dental clinic. The patient had been highly apprehensive throughout the procedure, even though 30 mg of Valium had been used.
   a. Inscription Meperidine 50 mg.
   b. Subscription Disp. 16 tabs
   c. Signatura 1 tab each 3-4 hrs.

3. A 34-year-old female has just undergone a quadrant of periosurgery including some osseous recontouring. She has tolerated the procedure well under nitrous oxide and claims that two aspirins take care of most of her headaches. She is on the whole a very cooperative patient and does not complain too much.
   a. Inscription Codeine phosphate 30 mg.
   b. Subscription Disp. 16 tabs
   c. Signatura 1 tab each 3-4 hrs.

4. A 56-year-old female has just undergone an apicoectomy. The patient was highly nervous throughout the procedure and constantly responded to even minor stimuli. She claims that aspirin, Darvon or codeine never work on her and that she wants strong medicine to take care of her discomfort.
   a. Inscription PENTAZOCINE 50 mg OR MEPERIDINE 50mg.
   b. Subscription DISP: 16 TABS.
   c. Signatura 1 TAB EACH 3-4 HRS.

5. A 23-year-old female has her husband call you the night following the removal of a mesioangular Class 1B impaction. You had, following surgery, given her a prescription for Empirin #3 (aspirin 325 mg, codeine 30 mg). The patient claims that she has taken three tablets within the last six hours and has had no relief of the pain. What do you suggest? 1 ASPIRIN @ EACH EMPIRIN #3

ANSWERS

1. a. Acetaminophen (or aspirin) 600 mg
   b. Disp: 32 tablets
   c. Take 2 tablets every 3-4 hours as necessary for pain

2. a. Meperidine 50 mg
   b. Disp: 16 tablets
   c. Take 1 tablet every 3-4 hours as necessary for pain

3. a. Codeine Phosphate 30 mg, or Propoxyphene with aspirin
   b. Disp: 16 tablets
   c. Take 1 tablet with 2 tablets Acetominophen (or aspirin) every 3-4 hours as necessary for pain

4. a. Pentazocine 50 mg, or Meperidine
   b. Disp: 16 tablets
   c. Take 1 tablet every 3-4 hours as necessary for pain

5. Have her take 1 aspirin with each Empirin #3.

SUMMARY OF REFERENCES AND LITERATURE CITED

_______________, **A Look at Prescriptions Dentists Write,** *Dental Economics,* Oct. 1979, pp. 69-72.

Cooper, S.A., Needle, S.E., Kruger, G.O., **Comparative Analgesic Potency of Aspirin and Ibuprofen,** *J. Oral Surgery,* vol. 35, November, 1977.

Hopkinson, J.H., et al.: **Acetaminophen (500 mg) vs. Acetaminophen (325 mg) for the relief of pain in episiotomy patients,** *Curr. Ther. Res.* 16:194 (March) 1974.

American Dental Association Council on Dental Therapeutics, **Accepted Dental Therapeutics,** Chicago, Ill. 60611 (new edition annually).

American Medical Association, **AMA Drug Evaluations** PSG, Acton, Mass. (revised every three years).

Baker, Charles E., ed., **Physician's Desk Reference,** Medical Economics Company, (revised annually).

Gerald N. Rotenberg, ed., **Compendium of Pharmaceuticals and Specialties,** Canadian Pharmaceutical Association,1979.

United States Pharmacopeial Convention, **United States Pharmacopeia Dispensing Information,** Rockville, Md., 1980 (revised every year).

United States Pharmacopeial Convention, **Dictionary of Drug Names,** Rockville, Md., 1980, 1981 (revised annually).

USEFUL ADDITIONAL SOURCES OF INFORMATION

Kastrup, E., Boyd, J., **Facts and Comparisons,** Facts & Comparisons, Inc., St. Louis, Mo. (monthly up-dates).

____________________, **FDA Drug Bulletin,** Department of Health Education and Welfare, Public Health Service, Food and Drug Administration, Rockville, Md. (published monthly).

Thomas J. Pullasch, ed., **Dental Drug Service Newsletter,** P.O. Box 1912, Glendale, California 91209 (published monthly).

Review of Literature Pertaining to the Use of the Phenylalkanoic Acid Derivatives Ibuprofen and Fenbufen in Dentistry

Cooper, S.A., Breen, J.F., Giuliani, R.L.: **Replicate studies comparing the relative efficacies of aspirin and indoprofen in oral surgery outpatients.** *J Clin Pharmacol* 19:151-159, 1979.

Cooper, S.A., Needle, S.E., Kruger, G.O.: **Comparative analgesic potency of aspirin and ibuprofen.** *J Oral Surg* 35:898-903, 1977.

Dionne, R.A.: **The pharmacological basis of pain control in dental practice: Analgesics.** *The Compendium on Continuing Education in General Dentistry* Vol. I, No. 3, May/June 1980.

Dionne, R.A., Campbell, R.L., Cooper, S.A., Hall, D.L., Buckingham, B.: **Inhibition of Postoperative Pain by Preoperative Administration of a Non-steroidal Anti-inflammatory Analgesic, Ibuprofen.** San Diego, American Pain Society, 1979.

Dionne, R.A., Cooper, S.A.: **Evaluation of preoperative ibuprofen for postoperative pain following third molar removal.** *Oral Surg* 45:851-856, 1978.

Henrikson, P.A., Tjernberg, A., Ahlstrom, U., Peterson, L.E.: **Analgesic efficacy and safety of fenbufen following surgical removal of a lower wisdom tooth: A comparison with acetylsalicylic acid and placebo.** *J Int Med Res* 7:107-116, 1979.

Lokken, P., Olsen, L., Brusaset, I., Norman-Pedersen, K.: **Bilateral surgical removal of impacted lower third molar teeth as a model for drug evaluation: A test with ibuprofen.** *Eur J Clin Pharmacol* 8:209-216, 1975.

McIntyre, B.A., Phelp, R.B., Inwood, M.J.: **Effect of ibuprofen on platelet function in normal subjects and hemophiliac patients.** *Clin Pharmacol Ther* 24:616-621, 1978.

Use this page for:

- **Summarizing prescriptions you will use for antibiotics**
- **Recording any additional information you may collect concerning the use of antibiotics**

Use this page for:

- **Summarizing prescriptions you will use for analgesics**
- **Recording any additional information you may collect concerning the use of analgesics**

Use this page for summarizing prescriptions for any additional drugs you may use frequently.

NOTES